Table of Contents

"If you tell the truth you don't have to remember anything."

-Mark Twain

Dedication

This book is dedicated to Uncle Steve, my wife, daughter and family both on Hawaii and the mainland for their support and, the thousands of patients that have, over the years, helped me to perfect my program and allowed me to help improve and save their lives. To the doctors that have referred to me, trusting me with their dear patients.

Introduction to the

Life Without Diabetes

George Kosmides

A Quick Quiz

Which of the following statements about Type 2 diabetes **do you believe to be correct**?

■ Type 2 diabetes is incurable and irreversible, but researchers are closing in on a cure soon.

■ Type 1 "childhood diabetes" diabetes is a purely a genetic problem. There's nothing you can do about it except take your insulin injections and hope for a new research breakthrough.

■ Pre diabetes, or insulin resistance, is a common blood sugar abnormality you can live with, and is considered "normal" so long as your glucose levels are controlled with medications.

■ Diabetes is no big deal. By closely monitoring your blood sugar and following your doctor's orders, you can enjoy a normal life and escape the horrific complications of diabetes like nerve damage, eventual blindness and loss of limbs through amputation- not to mention heart attack, stroke and Alzheimer's disease.

Amazingly, **all** of these statements are *false.*

Not only are all of these statements false, they're also extremely dangerous if you have diabetes or are on your way to developing it.

Now, I realize you've probably heard each of these pronouncements from numerous respected sources, such as your doctor, the American Diabetes Association (or ADA), the pharmaceutical industry, and the mainstream media. But every one of these popular untruths about diabetes is dead wrong, and I'll show you clinical research that disputes them all in my new book,

Helpful tip: To learn more about my book and the step-by-step diabetes-reversing plan it describes, visit www.georgekosmides.com *or if you seek to be a patient (I attend to both virtual and in office), please go to* georgekosmides.com

This book will also introduce you to actual patients who are a living proof that modern medicine's false statements about (and treatment of) diabetes are **expensive**, **complicated**, **risky** and designed for **failure**.

I can say with impunity that using the plan described in *The Life Without Diabetes in 90 Days*; I've **never** had a Type 2 patient who failed to get off their diabetes medications and related drugs **entirely**. And in almost every True Type 1 patient, I've been able to significantly reduce their insulin dose – usually by **85%** or **more!**

The Facts, Told Straight

- An estimated 285 million people[1], corresponding to **6.4%** of the world's adult population, were living with diabetes in 2010. The number is expected to grow to 438 million[2] by 2030, corresponding to **7.8%** of the adult population.

- While the global prevalence of diabetes[3] is **6.4%,** the prevalence varies from **10.2%** in the Western Pacific to **3.8%** in the African region. However, the African region is expected to experience the highest increase in the coming years.

- **70%** of the current cases of diabetes occur in low and middle income countries. With an estimated **50.8 million** people living with diabetes in India[4], followed by China[5] with **43.2 million** people.

- The largest age group currently affected by diabetes is between 40-59 years[6]. By 2030, this "record" is expected to move to the **60-79** age groups with an estimated number of **196 million** cases.

- Diabetes is one of the major causes of premature illness and death worldwide. Non-communicable diseases, including diabetes, account for **60%** of all deaths worldwide.

---

[1]World Diabetes Foundation, "Diabetes Facts," http://www.worlddiabetesfoundation.org/composite-35.htm (May 2011).

[2] http://www.worlddiabetesfoundation.org/composite-35.htm

[3] http://www.worlddiabetesfoundation.org/composite-35.htm

[4] Hindustan Times, "India, World Diabetes Capital," http://www.hindustantimes.com/India-world-diabetes-capital/Article1-245889.aspx (Sept. 2007)

[5] BBC News, "China Faces Diabetes Epidemic, Research Suggests," http://news.bbc.co.uk/2/hi/8587032.stm (May 2010).

[6] http://www.worlddiabetesfoundation.org/composite-35.htm.

If you didn't already know some of these facts, you can now understand how serious of an epidemic this really is. Having that knowledge, you might ask yourself a question that seems painfully simple: **Why aren't more physicians adopting this approach**, which so far has proved to be nothing but **successful**? The answer is disturbing, dangerous and just plain wrong.

The truth is being kept from us.

The fact that the medical establishment has failed to halt, contain and reverse the undeniably dreadful global diabetes epidemic is a colossal embarrassment to what I call the "System" or rather the "Business of Medicine" -- and indisputable evidence that something is very, very wrong with the current "official" approach to the diabetes problem.

Indeed, nearly everything the System is telling you about diabetes is both **false** and potentially **dangerous**. Recent unimpeachable scientific studies, from major peer-reviewed medical journals, have proven that Type 2 **and** pre-diabetes also known as insulin resistance, can be not only **halted**, but actually **reversed** without drugs, insulin or medical interventions. With this kind of scientific research published in respected medical journals, it seems obvious that the public is being lied to in an effort to cover up the facts about the underlying causes of diabetes as well as the questionable safety and undeniable ineffectiveness of the current medical treatments. The truth is that there are **easy**, **inexpensive**, **drug-free** ways to **halt** and, yes, **reverse** this condition.

Powerful forces in our society are in on these untruths, including the medical establishment (even their silence is condemnable), the pharmaceutical industry, insurance providers, food manufacturers, big Sugar, agribusiness lobbyists, and even the mainstream media (much of which depends on advertising from all of the aforementioned influences). In other words, there are a lot of people out there with wealth, influence and special interests, who are not interested in the greater wealth of humankind, but rather stand to profit immensely from the growing and surging diabetes explosion that is currently rocking the globe. The combined wealth, influence and sheer clout of these special interests are mind-boggling.

To be clear, I'm not suggesting that there's a conspiracy here. These are the simple fact that, as you'll read later on in the book, every party involved recognizes the staggering profit potential of the current and future situation, and as a result none of them wants to rock the boat-- regardless of how many people lose their lives in the process.

There is no real motivation for a cure, since "management", regardless of how ineffective it is, is the best for profits. **There is *no* profit in a cure!**

Are these criticisms too harsh?

Are they a too-quick rush to judgment?

Am I Paranoid?

I've been accused of all of these things and more, but can I assure you that naïvety is not my motivation. I'm tired of watching families be destroyed and lives thrown away all because the truth is not being told. The average Diabetic is left powerless, I wrote this book to help and change that…

Why, then, you might ask, am I so fervent about eliminating Type 2 Diabetes?

Two words: **Uncle Steve.**

Uncle Steve

Growing up, we all had a favorite uncle. Uncle Steve was mine. He was my hero, and nothing short of great. He was a talented guy - funny, well-liked by all, and a professional bowler to boot. He was so talented and a gifted bowler, he is one of a handful of people in the world to have scored perfect 300-point games in his short career. Not just one, but several!

For those of you that don't follow bowling, what this means is that he knocked down *all* of the pins each time he touched the ball in all the frames. In bowling, this is a huge deal - like winning the Olympic Gold Medal, or the Indy 500.

Uncle Steve was only **51** when he finally lost the battle to Type 2 diabetes, he suffered for several years before passing. His unbelievable bowling career was cut short, ending in his prime. Type 2 diabetes took him bit-by-bit. At the time, I was only able to watch my uncle's health fade, wanting to help as I know so many others have tried to, but not knowing how.

The joy of seeing Uncle Steve in his prime was replaced in his last years with sadness, worry and sympathy for the condition that diabetes left him in.

Uncle Steve lost the battle to diabetes on March 3rd, 1996. Again, <u>Needlessly</u>…

Uncle Steve's Legacy

The story I've just related is my "Why," "I built the passion to correct the irregularities involved when handling issues relating to this disease" this is my passion for the correction of this disease condition, Type 2 Diabetes.

As I came upon the information placed in this book, studying everything I could get my hands on and refining it over the last decade, I asked myself for a long time whether I should bring it forth to the general public, knowing that it may shake the very foundations of the healthcare establishment. Knowing fully well that I would constantly be under attack if this closely guarded information ever see the light of day.

There finally came a point, though, that I could not hold back any longer.

In becoming a doctor, I took an oath to help sick people get well. Knowing the information that I possess, I can't ignore that oath any longer! You deserve to have the full story about your disease.

My Medical Journey

I've worked in the medical industry long enough to witness the twisted politics, egotism and corruption, cover-ups and influence-peddling that guides its policy and practices. While there are many compassionate and devoted people in healthcare today, The System, which I'll explain more about in Chapter 2, is broken and can crush the spirit of even the most ethical medical professional. What I Call the "Business of Medicine."

And that's exactly what happened to me early in my clinical career. On my way to becoming a young physician, I worked in several clinics and couldn't help but notice that very little real healing was going on. I also witnessed the hugely restrictive political red tape that prevented creatively curious doctors from deviating from the official, recipe-like treatment protocols that merely "managed" symptoms while rarely addressing the underlying causes of the illness. This search for the underlying causes is the key to resolving the diseases, not merely treating it.

After an accident that nearly cost me my life, I shifted my studies to biological science, clinical nutrition and Chinese-based acupuncture and herbal medicine. I traveled throughout Asia, where I was taught acupuncture and herbal remedies, and also how to work with patients who were on drugs in order to safely help them to shift back to health. My craving for a vast and diverse array of knowledge was (and still is) immense, and I interned at clinics both in Asia and the United States. All the while, since 1991, I was also a practicing chiropractor. When I passed my certification exams in both areas, I was one of only a **handful of people** nationwide who had done so.

After graduation, I went to work at some of the most prestigious clinics in the world and was in constant company of some of the country's greatest practitioners. After several years in practice, I looked around, and I saw the same problems perpetuated in medical school, hospitals and in private practice.

I didn't want to reject conventional medicine completely. After all, I recognized that its treatments are appropriate in many instances, especially for acute and critical medical care patients. The best analogy that comes to mind is the MASH doctor. Excellent at removing shrapnel and mending bullet holes but, is he or she really trained to correct a Type 2 Diabetic. There is no training in healthy eating, nutrition. No, the training is just not there...

I had been interested in holistic health all along because I saw the importance of including both mind/body and emotional aspects of medicine in health care.

Physicians *do* want to heal, but most are <u>misinformed</u>.

While becoming a doctor, I came to the conclusion that I wanted a medical path that would train me in the art of true healing. This led me to focus my studies on wellness, or "real healing." This style, though, was no shortcut; working towards my doctorate in chiropractic, acupuncture, and clinical nutrition required over 5,000 plus hours and counting of training and study. That's more than what would have been required had I only chosen to get an MD, though these orientations are as different as night and day (as I'll soon explain).

What is Wellness?

<u>Wellness</u> [7] focuses on stimulating the body's inherent ability to heal and repair itself, using a <u>holistic approach and a minimum of surgery and drugs</u>[8]. This is the **true** tradition of the physician, hailing all the way back to <u>Hippocrates</u>[9], the ancient Greek referred to as "the father of modern medicine" and the first

---

[7] Wikipedia, "Wellness," http://en.wikipedia.org/wiki/Wellness_(alternative_medicine) (April 2011).

[8] New York Times Magazine, "Wellness," http://www.nytimes.com/2010/04/18/magazine/18FOB-onlanguage-t.html (April 2010).

[9] Wikipedia, "Hippocrates," http://en.wikipedia.org/wiki/Hippocrates (Oct. 2011)

advocate of natural medicine. Besides using a wide variety of natural remedies, our selected fraternity of wellness doctors emphasizes nutrition, proper nervous system function, prevention, lifestyle adjustments and patient education as pathways to body-mind health and well-being.

My experience speaks to over 5,000 hours of education and 20-plus years of healing in private practice. Rather than apply "band-aid" treatments for symptoms. Physicians like me who focus on **wellness** seek to correct the **<u>underlying causes of health problems</u>** so they can be resolved permanently. In doing so, we address the patient's psychological and emotional state *as well as* the physical. Our orientation to the healing process is summed up in the oath we take upon graduation:

- Above all else, do no harm -- and provide the most effective health care available with the least risk to patients at all times.
- Respect, recognize and promote the self-healing power of nature inherent in each individual.
- Identify and remove the causes of illness, rather than eliminating or suppressing symptoms.
- Educate and instill hope and encourage self-responsibility for health.
- Treat the whole person by considering all individual health factors and influences.
- Emphasize the principles of healthy living to promote well-being in order to prevent diseases in the individual, the community and our world.

Long ago, physicians took this <u>same oath</u>[10], but their Hippocratic Oath has been changed several times – especially in the modern era – to accommodate the use of today's drugs (many of which do indeed

---

[10]"The Hippocratic Oath," http://nktiuro.tripod.com/hippocra.htm (Sept. 1999).

cause harm) and to de-emphasize the long-honored focus on disease prevention[11] and patient education[12].

These changes were primarily economic considerations. What else might we expect when the pharmaceutical industry now has enormous influence on the curriculum of America's medical schools? Modern medicine, as a result, has become more of a business[13] and less of an art.

Backed by my rounded education from medical institutions around the world and a passionate desire to bring the art of unbiased care back to the field of medicine, I'm a licensed clinical practitioner for over 20 years now and have successfully treated thousands of patients. With this book, I hope to share this information which can save your life (**before** it's too late), with readers like you from around the world.

Life Without Diabetes

---

[11] Wikipedia, "Preventative Medicine," http://en.wikipedia.org/wiki/Preventive_medicine (Sept. 2011).

[12] Wikipedia, "Patient Education," http://en.wikipedia.org/wiki/Patient_education (June 2011).

[13] Neer, Joel, "Medical Schools and Drug Firm Dollars," http://www.npr.org/templates/story/story.php?storyId=4696316

Chapter 1: The Facts

I'm Dr. George Kosmides. I have over 20 years of experience with Type 2 diabetics. Losing Uncle Steve to diabetes (an experience I wrote about in the introduction) and watching the suffering he went through has supremely motivated me as a doctor to discover the best and most effective methods that get true *results*. With a keen knowledge of chemistry and the creation of an easy to follow system, I've created a plan that can have the blood sugar of those with Type 2 diabetes normalized in as little as 12 weeks. Yes, you read right- that's only three months.

How taking control of your diabetes treatment can help you reverse your disease *and* take your

life back.

In the United States, the Centers for Disease Control and Prevention (CDC)[14] have predicted[15] that **1 in 3** people will have Type 2 Diabetes by 2050 – up from **1 in 10** Americans who have this form of the disease today[16]. That is a staggering and dire statistic – but the truth is that it *doesn't* have to be that way. Whether you have just been diagnosed with Type 2 Diabetes or you have been living with it for some time, the clock is ticking and your disease may continue to progress if you don't have the right information and care at your disposal.

---

[14] Centers for Disease Control and Prevention, http://www.cdc.gov (Oct. 2011).

[15] CDC, "Successes and Opportunities for Population-Based Prevention and Control At A Glance 2011," http://www.cdc.gov/chronicdisease/resources/publications/AAG/ddt.htm (Aug. 2011).

[16] http://www.cdc.gov/chronicdisease/resources/publications/AAG/ddt.htm.

I know that I probably don't have to tell you this, but diabetes[17] is a medical condition caused by a lack of insulin in the body. There are two major forms of diabetes – Type 1 diabetes[18] (or diabetes mellitus), indicated by the body's lack of insulin and inability to produce it, and Type 2[19] (or diabetes insipidus) indicated by the body's resistance to the effects of insulin and sometimes even *reduced* production.

Not only is it the most common of the two types, but Type 2 Diabetes is also the most complicated version of the disease. It is triggered by a combination of factors; some of them, like family, history, and race are unchangeable and becoming less and less likely. While others, like obesity, inactivity, and lifestyle (your diet) are completely controllable. The major issue for Type 2 Diabetics is that they have developed a resistance to insulin in their bodies. What they might not know is that they also have the ability to influence their disease – positively and negatively. If you are a Type 2 diabetic, or pre-diabetic, and don't want to let this disease guide your life, **you must first take ownership of the role you can play** in advancing or **reversing** the disease.

There are a number of risk factors[20] for developing Type 2 Diabetes, which include:

- Being over 45

- Being overweight or obese

- Being of African American, Hispanic or Asian descent

- Being physically inactive

---

[17] Merriam-Webster, "Diabetes," http://www.merriam-webster.com/dictionary/diabetes (2011).

[18] Wikipedia, "Diabetes mellitus," http://en.wikipedia.org/wiki/Diabetes_mellitus (Oct. 2011).

[19] Wikipedia, "Diabetes insipidus," http://en.wikipedia.org/wiki/Diabetes_insipidus (Oct. 2011).

[20] Medline Plus, "Type 2 Diabetes Risk Factors," http://www.nlm.nih.gov/medlineplus/ency/article/002072.htm (June 2011).

- Having a family history of Diabetes

- Having high blood pressure and/or low levels of good cholesterol

- Lifestyle Choices

According to the Centers for Disease Control and Prevention's[21] 2011 National Diabetes Fact Sheet[22]:

- Nearly 26 million Americans have diabetes (that's 8.3% of the total population)

- Every 17-seconds someone new receives a Diabetes diagnosis, equaling 1.9 million new cases per year.

- It's estimated that another 79 million adults have pre-diabetes.

- Annually, the cost of diabetes adds up to about $174 billion!

Diabetes is also the seventh leading cause of death[23] in the United States. It is the leading cause of leg and foot amputations[24], kidney failure [25] and new cases of blindness[26] in adults UNDER the age of 75.

Why does the diabetes picture in America seem to be getting worse? Believe it or not, the answer lies in advances in medicine & technology. While it may seem counter-intuitive that advances in medicine are

---

[21] http://www.cdc.gov.

[22] CDC, "2011 National Diabetes Fact Sheet," http://www.cdc.gov/diabetes/pubs/pdf/ndfs_2011.pdf (June 2011).

[23] CDC, "Leading Causes of Death," http://www.cdc.gov/nchs/fastats/lcod.htm (Sept. 2011).

[24] National Diabetes Information Clearinghouse, "National Diabetes Statistics, 2011," http://diabetes.niddk.nih.gov/DM/PUBS/statistics/ (Feb. 2011).

[25] American Diabetes Association, "Diabetes Statistics," American Diabetes Association, "Diabetes Statistics," http://www.diabetes.org/diabetes-basics/diabetes-statistics/ (Jan. 2011).

[26] American Diabetes Association, "Diabetes Statistics," http://www.diabetes.org/diabetes-basics/diabetes-statistics/ (Jan. 2011).

actually *increasing* the prevalence of the disease, much of the increase in diagnosis of new cases of Type 2 Diabetes are a result of new technologies that enable earlier diagnosis and longer life through treatments designed to 'manage the disease and control progression.'

It must be noted, however, that living longer does not mean living better.

That's right. Many of today's medical professionals, the doctors you rely on to treat your disease, simply accept the fact that Type 2 diabetes is chronic[27]. Today's standard of care tries to increase longevity, sure, but it also has a little-to-no focus on the quality of life[28]. Their goal, from the instance of your diagnosis, is to manage your symptoms and delay the diagnosis of all the *other diseases* and the complications that could arise from being a Type 2 Diabetic.

Is that really what you want?

Complications associated with Type 2 Diabetes are far reaching. People living with diabetes and undergoing conventional care –which is intended simply **to manage symptoms and control progression** – often end up with secondary illnesses that are far more dangerous and deadly than the original diabetes. Even worse, these secondary illnesses often come with their own batch of medicines with side effects that can actually impact and worsen your diabetes.

This cannot possibly be a vicious cycle you want to be part of, can it?

[27]Merriam-Webster, "Chronic," http://www.merriam-webster.com/dictionary/chronic (Oct. 2011).

[28] Wikipedia, "Quality of life (healthcare)," http://en.wikipedia.org/wiki/Quality_of_life_(healthcare) (Aug. 2011).

According to the American Diabetes Association[29] and the 2011 National Diabetes Fact Sheet[30], the most common secondary disorders diagnosed in individuals following the conventional care method are the following:

1. **Heart Disease and Stroke** – noted as the cause of death on 68% of diabetes-related death certificates in 2004.

2. **High Blood Pressure** – 67% of adult diabetics (aged 20+) had blood pressure greater than or equal to 140/90 or used prescription medications to control hypertension.

3. **Blindness** – the leading cause of new cases of blindness[31] for adults aged 20-74; 28.5% of individuals within 40-years or older with diabetes (4.2 million) were diagnosed with diabetic retinopathy between 2005 and 2008.

4. **Kidney Disease.** Diabetes is the leading cause of kidney failure and accounts for 44% of new cases annually.

5. **Nervous System Disease -** 60-70% of people with diabetes have mild-to-severe forms of nervous system damage.

6. **Amputation** – more than 60% of non-traumatic lower-limb amputation occur in people with diabetes.

7. **Dental disease** – periodontal disease is more common in people with diabetes than in non-diabetics.

---

[29] American Diabetes Association, "American Diabetes Association," http://www.ada.org," (Oct. 2011).

[30] http://www.cdc.gov/diabetes/pubs/pdf/ndfs_2011.pdf

[31] http://www.diabetes.org/diabetes-basics/diabetes-statistics/

8. **Pregnancy complications** – gestational diabetes occurs in between 3 and 10% of all pregnancies.

And let's not forget one of the deadliest- **cancer**. Recent medical studies, such as this one[32] from 2005, also show that people with diabetes are at increased for certain cancers. Diabetics are **twice** as likely to be diagnosed with liver, pancreas or endometrial cancer. They are 20-50% more likely to develop colorectal[33], breast and bladder cancer.

Now, to be honest, there has been some debate about whether or not a *direct* correlation between diabetes treatments and increased cancer risk. There is a significant number of shared risk factors[34], as cancer and diabetes become more common as people age; increased weight gain, poor diets, and smoking have all been shown as potential causes for both cancer and diabetes. Both groups of patients can also have off-kilter metabolisms, and be overweight or obese. As you can see the links are there, but whether the two are directly related or not is still in the waiting to be scientifically determined.

The more important question here is whether or not **you're willing to *risk* the wait**.

Another important thing to know is that none of these secondary disorders are written in the stars. None of these dangerous outcomes *have* to be a part of your future. **You** have the power to **take control** of

---

[32] PubMed, "Possible participation of advanced glycation end products in the pathogenesis of colorectal cancer in diabetic patients," http://www.ncbi.nlm.nih.gov/pubmed/15823719 (2005).

[33] Journal of the National Cancer Institute, "Prospective Study of Adult Onset Diabetes Mellitus (Type 2) and Risk of Colorectal Cancer in Women," http://jnci.oxfordjournals.org/content/91/6/542.full (Sept. 1998).

[34] PubMed, "Diabetes and Cancer," http://www.ncbi.nlm.nih.gov/pubmed/19620249 (Dec. 2009).

your disease and **take back** your life. An added bonus to actively engaging in how your disease is treated is that you'll not only feel better, live healthier and possibly even longer, but that you'll save money while doing it, too.

Speaking of the money…

- **$174 billion** was spent for treating diagnosed diabetes in the US in 2007 **alone**. This breaks down to **$116 billion** for direct medical costs (medicines, supplies, doctor visits, surgeries, etc.).

- **$58 billion** for indirect costs (disability, work loss, premature mortality).

- **$18 billion** in expenses for undiagnosed diabetes,

- **$25 billion** for adults with prediabetes[35]

- **$623 million** for gestational diabetes and you've got the United States' annual expenditures for diabetes treatment adding up to a whopping **$218 billion**!

It is also estimated that the out-of-pocket expenses for *insured* diabetics is about **$6,000 to $10,000** annually!

Take a minute - just 60 seconds, and think about how many things you could do if you **didn't have** that expense.

---

[35] Wikipedia, "Prediabetes," http://en.wikipedia.org/wiki/Prediabetes (Sept 2011).

Though the mainstream medical and pharmaceutical industries may say otherwise, developing one or more of these complications is *not* inevitable. In fact, **there are ways you can help prevent and reverse Type 2 diabetes.**

Like a lot of other diseases, Type 2 diabetes creeps in slowly but the impacts – when untreated or improperly treated – can be lifelong. Despite what you may have been told, there is a *real* solution out there for Type 2 Diabetics. There are *real* options – that don't rely on adding more meds to your prescription or changing doses. There are steps you can take to get your life back **now,** and live a longer, happier, healthier life **free** of Type 2 Diabetes and its related complications in the future.

We will go into more specifics later on in the book, but the items listed below, when properly implemented, are *key* to your **improvement.**

- **Eat Right** – The American Diabetes Association[36] recommends cutting back on meal sizes and going for smaller portions, drinking calorie-free drinks (but not Splenda - and I will tell you why), eating low-fat versions of regular foods, eating more grilled or baked lean meats, eating more vegetables and cutting back on high-fat dressings, toppings or condiments. (My menu plan will make it so very simple)…

- **Exercise** – More than **80%** of people with Type 2 Diabetes are overweight or obese. Carrying excess weight – especially around the abdomen – greatly increases the risk for Diabetes. Reducing your body weight even as little as **10%** can have a positive impact on the body's

---

[36] http://www.ada.org.

ability to process/absorb insulin. A basic, easy, not fanatical way to improve your circumstances. Body fat reduction is even more important…

- **Get more rest** – A <u>recent study</u> [37] published in the May 2010 *Journal of Clinical Endocrinology and Metabolism* showed that getting an inadequate night's sleep (less than 8 hours) can increase insulin resistance, consequently increasing the risk of Type 2 diabetes.

- **Stop Smoking** – Smokers are **50-90%** more likely to develop diabetes than non-smokers. Smoking can harm the pancreas, increase blood sugar levels, and impair the body's ability to use the insulin it does manage to produce, as shown in a <u>1993 study.</u>

I know, a World of Facts

I understand that this information is a lot to process. There are a lot of studies and research out there to be absorbed. What's more, many doctors have been trained to utilize and follow a 'standard of care' that includes a combination of drug therapies that manage symptoms and help to control disease progression. But when it comes down to it, why would you want your disease to progress at all? Why not try to stop it instead?

You aren't the doctor. You don't have to know what to do. But you do have to know that your actions (and inaction) play a major role in your Type 2 Diabetes and that **you** have as much power as your doctor – if not *more* – in choosing your treatment path. In *Life Without Diabetes in 90 Days,* I never

---

[37] Journal of Clinical Endocrinology & Metabolism, "A Single Night of Partial Sleep Deprivation Induces Insulin Resistance in Multiple Metabolic Pathways in Healthy Subjects," http://jcem.endojournals.org/content/95/6/2963.abstract (June 2010).

settle for managing the disease, and I don't expect you to either. I also understand that no two people with diabetes are the same and that **they cannot be treated the same**. Life Without Diabetes in 90 Days uses state-of-the-art diagnostic tools and investigative diagnostic tests (these can be mailed to you or reviewed if you have them already) to **accurately assess** where your disease is at and how best to **reverse** it. It is an integrated approach that will produce results and allow you to re-claim your overall well-being, and allow you to live a happier, healthier, and longer diabetes-free life.

I have over 20 years of clinical experience treating diabetic patients and will help you to:

- **Learn why your insulin and other drug therapies might actually be the cause of many of your diabetic complications.**
- **Control your blood sugar levels, treat complications and achieve overall wellness.**
- **Practice a safe and natural ways to lose weight, eliminate drugs and reduce other diabetic complications.**
- **Save money by reducing your need for medications and related diabetes treatment supplies.**

Think back to a time before you had your Type 2 Diabetes diagnosis. Remember how great it felt not even knowing what a blood glucose level was, or having to worry about it in your day-to-day life? Remember what it was like to have enough energy to last all day long? Now, imagine all of the things you would do if you could go back to that!

With the help of *Life Without Diabetes in 90 Days* you can **reverse** your disease. You can **rediscover** good health and wellness.

Don't wait another day. Read the book, follow its simple steps and you too can be free of Type 2 Diabetes in 90 days, period.

In need of some extra support on your journey to recovery? Check out our diabetes Skype group[38] today! Or email me at Info@leanbodyacademy.com and my web address @ www.georgekosmides.com

Chapter 2

Type 2 Diabetes Untruths: Unraveling the Workings of the System

I've been a licensed clinical practitioner for over 20 years and have treated thousands of patients. My eclectic training and background allow me a unique perspective on today's serious health problems – and the solutions that the medicine and pharmaceutical companies don't want you to know. There is one truth out there that I think is incredibly important to share:

Virtually all of today's chronic and degenerative diseases are **preventable** and **reversible**.

Why then are these kinds of epidemics occurring?

---

[38] http://www.georgekosmides.com

A corporate takeover of the medical profession had shifted the role of physicians from serving as healers, (the word "doctor"[39] actually means "to teach") to a much more corrupt role as distributors of pharmaceutical drugs or worse, with little real focus on education.

There are now leagues of doctors educated by pharmaceutical reps (you usually see them in medical complexes, dressed in business suits, pulling their drugs in an expensive suitcase). They have no real medical training at all.

Again, for these people trained in the art business and **not** medical science, it does not appear to be in "their" best interest to have a *truly healthy* population.

The Untruths, Debunked

So what exactly is the System not telling you about diabetes, or should I say, how are they misleading you? Let us count the ways:

Un-Truth #1: "We're not exactly sure what causes pre-diabetes and Type 2 diabetes."

Some experts attribute it to obesity. Others say it's our modern sedentary lifestyle. Still, others blame the patients themselves, implying they are lazy and slothful. Rarely does the System place the responsibility

---

[39] Online Etymology Dictionary, "Doctor," http://www.etymonline.com/index.php?term=doctor (2011).

where it deserves to be: on the foods you've been taught to crave. What you're not being told is how terrible they are for your health- how they constitute **a** causal link[40] to this terrible disease.

The truth: The global pandemic of Type 2 diabetes and pre-diabetes is caused **directly** by our **modern diet** and its highly-processed foods[41]. These include high-carbohydrate/low-nutrient junk, overly-processed refined foods and metabolism-distressing ingredients such as high-fructose corn syrup, Trans fats, refined vegetable oils and artificial sweeteners. Factor in hidden allergies to wheat and other substances (which stress and weaken the human immune system) and a catastrophic absence of high-fiber, nutrient-dense whole foods[42] – fresh fruits and vegetables, whole grains and beans, and humanely-raised, hormone-free meat, eggs, fish, and dairy products and you have a perfect recipe for diabetes.

The reason: If this truth were widely revealed, and if public health officials openly condemned this diabetes-causing diet, the economic repercussions would be devastating for the giant agribusiness corporations that grow the raw materials for these commercial "**food-like products**," a term I prefer because much of what's produced doesn't qualify as real "whole food" in my book.

The truth would also hit the manufacturers and marketers who stock these products in our supermarkets, the supermarkets themselves, and the media, which thrives on the advertising revenue that these

---

[40] Science Direct, "Evidence for a Food Additive as a Cause of Ketosis-Prone Diabetes," http://www.sciencedirect.com/science/article/pii/S0140673681910485 (Aug. 2003).

[41] Diabetic Lifestyle, "Red Meat and Processed Options Shown to Increase Type 2 Diabetes Risk,"http://www.diabeticlifestyle.com/diabetes-news/type-2-diabetes/red-meat-processed-options-shown-increase-type-2-diabetes-risk" (Aug. 2011).

[42] Health Sentinel, "High Glycemic and Low Fiber Foods Associated with Diabetes,"http://www.healthsentinel.com/joomla/index.php?option=com_content&view=article&id=342:high-glycemic-and-low-fiber-foods-associated-with-diabetes&catid=5:original&Itemid=24 (Aug. 2004).

26

products generate. I assure you that unimaginable sums of money are being generated as diabetes develops and spreads.

Were the medical community to point a finger directly at the foods and beverages causing today's avalanche of Type 2 and pre-diabetes in unaware adults and defenseless children, it would trigger a massive cry from the billion-dollar industries involved, as well as a lobbying barrage more colossal than Washington and other capitals around the world have ever seen. Placing the blame on obesity, lack of exercise or the patients themselves is a deceitful distraction from the true cause. That the medical and scientific communities are instrumental in this deceit — or, just as worse, remain silent when they have a chance to speak out — is nothing short of malpractice.

Untruth #2: "The American diet (like our medical system) is the best in the world."
We've been conditioned to believe that our supermarkets and dinner tables are the envy of the world, and that our doctors and hospitals are the best on the planet.

The truth: All of our food-related government watchdog agencies, which are supposed to be protecting our health, are obstructed by contradictory goals and objectives, as well as by massive special-interest lobbying. This includes the USDA (responsible for the safety of agricultural products), the FDA (for effectiveness and safety of pharmaceutical drugs), the EPA (for environmental quality) and the FTC (for the quality of broadcast programming and advertising). Literally, billions of US tax dollars in the form of federal agriculture subsidies are pumped into price supports for sugar, corn, wheat, soybeans and feedlot beef – the raw materials from which many diabetes-causing food products are made. All the while, almost nothing goes to small farmers struggling to raise organic fruits, vegetables, and livestock.

27

US agricultural capacity, which politicians love to boast about, is based on volume, not quality. In actual fact, America's bountiful harvests are the result of copious applications of synthetic fertilizers, herbicides, pesticides, growth hormones, antibiotics and a host of other dubious chemicals that are linked[43] to numerous health problems in our population. Many studies show that these agricultural chemicals depress the body's immune system, compromise the liver (our most important organ for detoxification) and attack the beta cells of the pancreas (which produce insulin). These facts are well known, but the scientific community overall remains hauntingly silent.

Just one example: 83 active pesticide ingredients[44] known and shown to cause cancer in animals or humans are still in use today.

The reason: Cleaning up our agricultural system would result in hundreds of billions of dollars in lost profits for every industry involved.

As for the superlative quality of our food and medical systems, both are factual falsities.

FACTS

- The US is 33rd out of 195 nations in infant mortality

_____

[43] Current Opinion in Neurology, "Pesticides and Parkinsonism: is there an etiological link?" http://journals.lww.com/co.neurology/Abstract/2000/12000/Pesticides_and_Parkinsonism__is_there_an.13.aspx (Dec. 2000).

[44] Infinite Health Resources, "Pesticide Statistics," http://www.infinitehealthresources.com/Store/Resource/Article/1-35/2/189.html (Jan. 2006).

28

- 47th in life expectancy of 225 countries

- 14th in heart disease mortality.

- 16th highest in the incidence of breast cancer

- 9th in cancer deaths,

and we have nearly **four times the incidence of diabetes compared to the world average**.

When it comes to the incidence of preventable diseases, the US is 17th in the world[45], right behind Portugal; which means it's healthier there than it is here. There is, though, one health statistic that we do lead every other nation on earth in: obesity.

Untruth #3:

"Type 1 diabetes is a genetic phenomenon, and there isn't much we can do about it."

In this case, the **mainstream public is being lied to, period**. This untruth attempts to convince people that Type 1 diabetes is an autoimmune disease in which the body's immune system destroys its own insulin-producing beta cells. Once the cells are wiped out, the doctors would say, "they're gone forever," and the patient must then rely on lifelong insulin injections.

The truth: Fascinating new research is questioning with new research.

---

[45] United Press International, "US Ranks Last in Preventable Deaths," http://www.upi.com/Health_News/ 2011/09/23/US-ranks-last-in-preventable-deaths/UPI-36321316827953/?spt=hs&or=hn (Sept. 2011).

For one thing, Type 1 diabetes is rapidly rising right along with Type 2. Relatively rare 200 years ago, Type 1 is now twice as common [46] among children as it was in the 1980s and five times greater in prevalence than it was after the World War II. Epidemiologists said that[47] the incidence of Type 1 diabetes is 1000% higher than it was 100 years ago.

How can this be true if genetics are responsible? Human genes don't change that rapidly, but our lifestyle and environment certainly do. One emerging theory is that Type 1 isn't an autoimmune malfunction at all, but rather the immune system disposing of beta cells[48] that have been damaged in some way – by a virus, environmental toxins or food chemicals, including Alloxan in white flour and bread (read more about this beta-cell killer in *The Life Without Diabetes in 90 Days* meal plan).

Research is also disproving the "once they're gone, they're gone" theory about beta cells. Preliminary studies show that certain foods and supplements may indeed regenerate beta cells in the pancreas so that they can produce insulin again. Other nutrients have been found to strengthen the remaining beta cells in Type 2 diabetics so that they can once again produce insulin naturally.

Finally, easy lifestyle modifications described in *Life Without Diabetes* can increase the body's insulin sensitivity, allowing Type 1 patients to reduce their insulin dosage dramatically.

---

[46] Govita Tonunda, "Diabetes, a Worldwide Epidemic," http://www.upi.com/Health_News/2011/09/23/US-ranks-last-in-preventable-deaths/UPI-36321316827953/?spt=hs&or=hn (July 2011).

[47] American Diabetes Association, "The Rise of Childhood Type 1 Diabetes in the 21st Century," http://diabetes.diabetesjournals.org/content/51/12/3353.short (April 2002).

[48] Wikipedia, "Beta cell," http://en.wikipedia.org/wiki/Beta_cell (July 2011).

My Type 1 diabetes patient, James F is a good example. He was able to cut his dose by **80%** by following this book. Significant insulin reductions like these allow patients to avoid diabetic complications later in life.

An extreme case, resolved

A new patient, (at the time my office managers husband) walked into my office with blood sugar level, of **771**. After following the principles in Life Without Diabetes, his average blood sugar level dropped down to **130 to 105.** Again, not overnight but… It did drop… Without anything extreme.

My mission to get past the hype in order to help you reach true wellness has been successful, as proven in this case and many others.

The reason: Call me cynical, but I'm not seeing any mainstream curiosity about reviving the strength of beta cells, or how inside these cells are the Islets of Langerhans[49] – or about getting Type 1 patients on lower doses of insulin (even though this could greatly improve their outcomes). The global insulin market is currently worth **$3 billion** and growing at **14% annually**. Need I say more?

Un-Truth #4: "Managing your blood sugar with drugs is the most successful treatment for Type 2 and pre-diabetes."

---

[49]Wikipedia, "Islets of Langerhans," http://en.wikipedia.org/wiki/Islets_of_Langerhans (Sept. 2011).

The truth: I'll discuss this misconception in more detail in another special report I've written (*Mistakes Doctors Are Making with Diabetes*). It will suffice to say that diabetes drugs are unnecessary for a majority of pre-diabetes and Type 2 patients. The only instance in which I even *consider* drugs for these patients is in emergency situations, and "Even then, I keep on reducing the dosages as soon as possible". Lab testing will confirm the correction. Not only are they unnecessary, but many of these drugs are dangerous -- and has been proven so for years.

Vigilant glucose monitoring does nothing[50] to prevent diabetic complications, and this is being proven conclusively. Furthermore, self-monitoring of blood glucose (SMBG) encourages the same bad diet and poor lifestyle habits that allowed the disease to get a foothold in the first place. In my office, I recommend self-monitoring but also supply proper tools and education that is just not in today's Diabetic arsenal.

The reason: Glucose monitoring is very useful in Type 1 patients who take insulin – and occasionally for certain Type 2 patients under supportive care and that are prone to low blood sugar (hypoglycemia)[51], particularly those on sulfonylurea drugs. But in general, Type 2 diabetes can be managed effectively with the easy diet, nutrition and exercise you'll discover in this Life Without Diabetes book.

---

[50] Informed Health Online, "Type 2 diabetes: Does self-monitoring urine and blood glucose levels have benefits for people who do not inject insulin?" http://www.informedhealthonline.org/type-2-diabetes-does-self-monitoring-urine-and-blood-glucose-levels.671.en.html (July 2011).

[51] PubMed Health, "Hypoglycemia," http://www.ncbi.nlm.nih.gov/pubmedhealth/PMH0001423/ (June 2011).

Two studies published in the British Medical Journal confirmed this. The first study[52] split a group of newly diagnosed Type 2 patients into equal self-monitoring and no-monitoring groups. After 12 months, the diabetes (as measured by hemoglobin A1C testing) was no better in the self-monitoring group. The second study [53] divided a separate population of Type 2 patients into three groups: no monitoring, moderate monitoring, and intense monitoring. Not only did self-monitoring fail to improve diabetes control, but it also cost more. More importantly, they found that monitoring actually decreased the patients' quality of life.

Despite this well-published research, most doctors and the ADA continue to recommend self-monitoring. One has to wonder if the cost of test strips and glucose monitors has anything to do with this.

And now, the biggest untruth of them all.

Untruth #5:

"Type 2 diabetes can be managed successfully, but it isn't reversible." This is the biggest untruth of them all – and the most damaging. Why? **Because it keeps patients powerless and dependent on the System**. It turns them into cash cows to be regularly "milked" by the diabetes Type 1 and Type 2

---

[52]PubMed Central, "Impact of self monitoring of blood glucose in the management of patients with non-insulin treated diabetes: open parallel group randomized trial," http://www.ncbi.nlm.nih.gov/pubmedhealth/PMH0001423/ (July 2007).

[53]PubMed Central, "Frequency of blood glucose monitoring in relation to glycemic control: observational study with diabetes database," http://www.ncbi.nlm.nih.gov/pmc/articles/PMC28155/ (July 1999).

industry, with purveyors of junky, diabetes-causing food products continuing to create more future patients.

The truth: **Many scientific research proves that both pre-diabetes and Type 2 can be reversed with a few easy diet, nutrition and lifestyle modifications**, just like those presented in this Life Without Diabetes book.

For example, in 1982, nutritional researcher, Kerin O'Dea[54] restored [55] a group of severely diabetic Australian aboriginal men to good health simply by getting them off the typical Western diet of refined carbohydrates and its accompanying sedentary lifestyle (the two major causes of Type 2).

No medication or insulin was required.

The men in the study were badly overweight and insulin-resistant, with seriously elevated cholesterol, triglycerides and high blood pressure (all major risk factors for heart attack and stroke). In short, they were headed for a shortened lifespan with miserable complications, including gangrene, blindness, heart failure, various cancers and amputations of digits and limbs caused by nerve damage.

After just seven weeks on her plan, Dr. O'Dea drew blood samples from the men and discovered these dramatic changes:

---

[54]University of South Australia, "Professor Kerin O'Dea," http://www.unisanet.unisa.edu.au/staff/Homepage.asp?Name=kerin.o'dea (2011).

[55] Department of Medicine, St. Vincent's Hospital, "Preventable chronic disease in Indigenous Australian populations: the need for a comprehensive national approach,"

34

- Blood triglycerides, glucose and cholesterol levels had plummeted into the healthy range.

- Blood pressure had dropped significantly and normalized.

- The men had lost an average of nearly 20 pounds each.

In Dr. O'Dea's own words, **"All of the metabolic abnormalities of Type 2 diabetes were either greatly improved or completely normalized."** **The markers for diabetes and heart disease were** *completely* **gone!**

The reason: This discovery, in my view, was as significant as some of the most famous in medical history, ranking right up there with Lister (sterilization), Pasteur (germ theory), Fleming (antibiotics), and other medical super-heroes. Like the work of these brilliant medical pioneers, O'Dea's discovery could have prevented unnecessary suffering and saved millions of lives had it been heeded and adopted in mainstream practice. Instead, her research got buried because of medical politics and food industry pressure.

Other research has confirmed Dr. O'Dea's finding's regarding the prevention and reversal of Type 2 and pre-diabetes:

- In 1984, the journal *Diabetes* reported on a clinical study[56] done at the University of Vermont College of Medicine proving that increased physical activity boosts cell sensitivity to insulin – thus reversing the insulin resistance that is the precursor to (and underlying cause of) Type 2 diabetes. These findings were

---

[56] Diabetes Care Journal, "Role and Management of Exercise in Diabetes Mellitus, "http://care.diabetesjournals.org/content/11/2/201 (1988).

confirmed by a 2003 study published in *Diabetes Care* demonstrating that sedentary adults who simply added walking to their daily routine cut their risk of developing insulin resistance (pre-diabetes), even if they didn't lose any weight.

■ Researchers at the UCLA School of Medicine found that 50% of Type 2 patients were able to <u>reverse their diabetes in just three weeks</u>[57] by making small changes in their diet and adding moderate exercise. According to lead researcher Dr. Christian K. Roberts, "The study shows, contrary to common belief, that Type 2 diabetes and metabolic syndrome can be reversed solely through lifestyle changes."

■ In 2001, the New England Journal of Medicine <u>published research</u>[58] showing that even the easiest dietary changes can reduce the risk of developing Type 2 diabetes by nearly 60%. Subsequent studies (which included switching to the delicious, healthful foods you'll discover in Life Without Diabetes[59]) improved this reduction in diabetes to greater than 95%.

■ In 2001, the <u>largest study</u> [60] ever conducted to test the ability of diet and exercise to prevent pre-diabetes from turning into full-blown Type 2 proved to be a smashing success. Doctors at 27 medical centers around the country enrolled 3,234 people and assigned them to receive the drug Metformin (Glucophage), a placebo, or a lifestyle program involving classes and coaches who kept track of their progress. After three years, the lifestyle program cut the participants' risk of developing diabetes

---

[57] News Medical "<u>Study finds short-term lifestyle changes improve health even without major weight loss</u>," http://www.news-, medical.net/news/2006/01/10/15308.aspx (Jan 2006).

[58] New England Journal of Medicine, "Diet, Medicine, and the Risk of Type 2 Diabetes Mellitus in Women," <u>http://geocities.ws/mim_ebm/DMwomen.pdf</u> (2001).

[59]Kosmides, Dr. George, "<u>georgekosmides.com</u> (Oct. 2011).

[60]Diabetes Care Journal, "Effect of Metformin in Pediatric Patients With Type 2 Diabetes," <u>http://care.diabetesjournals.org/content/25/1/89.full</u> (Aug. 2001).

by more than **50%** -- a much better result than Metformin provided. "I don't see this as out of reach for the 10 million people who are at high risk for diabetes," said the study's director (that figure today is closer to 60 million Americans alone).

■ A Duke University Medical School study[61] found that Type 2 diabetics who reduced their consumption of carbohydrates achieved better blood sugar control and more effective weight loss than those who went on a typical calorie-restricted diet. After just six months, the low-carb group had lower hemoglobin A1C results, lost more weight with **95%** being able to reduce or even completely *eliminate* their diabetes medications. Plus, as little as a **five percent** weight loss –about 10 pounds for most people in the study – reduced the risk of diabetes by **58%**. Numbers like that are both truly inspiring and remarkable. "It's easy" says Eric Westman, MD, director of Duke's Lifestyle Medicine Program and lead author of the study. "If you cut out the carbohydrates, your blood sugar goes down, and you lose weight, which lowers your blood sugar even further. It's a one-two punch."

Chapter 3: A New Hope

The Brave Few

Here's an example of some of the positive steps that have been taken by a few brave souls in recent years, despite the overwhelming pressures of the mainstream medical, pharmaceutical and agricultural

---

[61]PubMed Central, "A low-carbohydrate, ketogenic diet to treat type 2 diabetes," http://www.ncbi.nlm.nih.gov/pmc/articles/PMC1325029/ (Dec. 2003).

industries, as well as the mainstream media. In 2009 the Institute of Medicine published a scathing investigative report[62] about the billions that get poured into wooing doctors into using their brand of drugs by pharmaceutical companies; of course, at this time period it is doubtful that true legislation will come about to fix this, but it is at least a positive step towards awareness.

Another instance is of research hospitals at some of Harvard Medical Schools closing the immense amount of funding received from pharmaceutical companies after protests from students unaware of the fact that their professors were not providing[63] the unbiased education that they signed up for.

These were reasonable actions, I thought, but the fact is that **none** of these things should be *happening in the first place*.

In recent times, I've witnessed the amazing shift in the general conscience of people, realizing for the first time the power of the body to heal itself if we just give it a chance. I was disturbed that conventional medicine was all but ignoring this near-miraculous power in its midst; and quite often obstructing it with drugs, misinformation, and interventions that are health suppressive. I'm telling you all this so you'll be reassured that I'm not a tree-hugging medical heretic, when I say you're being lied to about diabetes. You are.

---

[62] Institute of Medicine, "Conflict of Interest in Medical Research, Education and Practice," http://www.iom.edu/Reports/2009/Conflict-of-Interest-in-Medical-Research-Education-and-Practice.aspx (Apr. 2009).

[63] New York Times, "Harvard Teaching Hospitals Cap Outside Pay," http://www.nytimes.com/2010/01/03/health/research/03hospital.html (Jan. 2010).

I've been a licensed clinical practitioner for over 20 years and have treated thousands of patients. My eclectic training and background allow me a unique perspective on today's serious health problems – and the solutions that the medicine and pharmaceutical companies don't want you to know.

Actress Halle Berry Reverses Her Type 1 Diabetes

Another big misconception about diabetes is that Type 1 is hopelessly irreversible. This assumption may not be entirely correct. Promising new research in which dead insulin-producing beta cells have been revived and regenerated is making some scientists doubt this assumption. You'll read more about this in Life Without Diabetes[64]. Then there is the inexplicable mystery of how Academy Award-winning actress Halle Berry reversed her Type 1 diagnosis[65].

"One day, I simply passed out, and I didn't wake up for seven days, which is obviously very serious." That was how a leading actress found out she had Type 1 diabetes at age 39. When she awoke, doctors told her she'd need daily insulin injections for the rest of her life to avoid passing out again. Berry was an improbable diabetic: no family history, slim and athletically active. But she accepted her diagnosis and treatment plan -- and even became a celebrity spokesperson for the insulin manufacturer Novo Nordisk.

Then came her "miracle cure." She changed her diet, cutting out sugar, desserts, junk

---

[64] georgekosmides.com ask for updates here.

[65] The Daily Mail, "Halle Berry: My Battle with Diabetes," http://www.dailymail.co.uk/health/article-371528/Halle-Berry-My-battle-diabetes.html (Dec. 2005).

food and refined carbohydrates. "I started to eat loads of wonderful fresh vegetables, chicken, fresh fish, and pasta." She also upped her activity level, doing yoga daily, rollerblading and working out in the gym. "I needed to pay attention to everything that could affect my blood sugar level, including diet, and exercise and stress," she said. Then, in October 2007, she told reporters: "I've managed to wean myself off insulin, so now I like to put myself in the Type 2 category." Her statement was met with universal skepticism. "Impossible!" medical journalists

responded. "It must have been a misdiagnosis," diabetes specialists concluded. ABC News ran an article stating: "Despite her claims to the contrary, Halle Berry did not cure herself of Type 1 diabetes for one easy reason – Type 1 diabetes is incurable."

You'd think doctors would have been eager to study the actress more closely, in an open-minded attempt to see if her experience might, in some way, help other Type 1 patients. But the diabetes community wasn't interested. Meanwhile, Halle Berry continues to live a happy, healthy and drug-free life without diabetes.

Why aren't more doctors getting the message?

Because there is no real motivation. I don't say any of this wig glee…

Until now, a handful of doctors have known that diet and lifestyle modification might improve diabetes, but they have had little experience and even less time to educate their patients. Given the amount of time needed for adequate patient education and ongoing support and motivation, the preference for a quick fix involving drugs is far more convenient. Sadly, profit-driven insurance providers have turned physicians into business people.

lifewithoutdiabetesbook.com

This is why I wrote "Life Without Diabetes." It **empowers** you to use education, the most potent medicine on earth, to help you improve and even reverse your diagnosis. Step-by-step and day-by-day, you'll read and learn how to heal your diabetic or pre-diabetic condition, balance your blood sugar, stabilize and rebuild your insulin production, lose the weight that aggravates your condition *without* dieting, strengthen your cardiovascular system, protect yourself from diabetic complications, and **lengthen your life**!

Life Without Diabetes has succeeded with my patients, and it will help you succeed, too. I've never had a Type 2 patient that I haven't been able to move **completely off medications**. Nor have I had a Type 1 diabetic for whom I haven't **significantly reduced** their insulin.

It just makes sense.

Insulin does not "cure," so what is there to do?

If you are on an insulin merry-go-round, you're gaining weight, feeling cold, or feeling your vision failing (or even worse, you may have several of the side effects already happening at once). **Don't lose heart.**

You may be a candidate for a cure and a healthy, hopeful new life.

A word to the wise...

Please understand this: if you're on insulin, keep taking it, no one is going to tell you to stop. Your testing results, as they improve or get worse over time, will dictate the reduction or increase.

The **only** thing that matters is your desire to live a **healthy life- a quality life,** free of constant monitoring of your blood sugars, free from the need to constantly monitor your diet - in short , **your desire to be whole again.**

You can achieve this with the tools in this Life Without Diabetes book[66].

My promise to you and to Uncle Steve (if he were here)

You can significantly improve your current condition without medications, daily finger sticks, "lap-band" surgery, stupid weight-loss dieting, ridiculous exercise or a strict food regimen.

In *"Life Without Diabetes",* you'll eat delicious food, shed pounds without trying, and nurture your body back to health with step-by-step instructions that are easy to follow.

---

[66]georgekosmides.com.

The best news is that my book contains an easy, natural, inexpensive and **proven** way out of today's distressing diabetes conundrum. To discover exactly how it achieves this goal, please read this book; follow the meal plan and follow-up with your progress on the Life Without Diabetes[67].

---

[67]georgekosmides.com.

See What Our Patients Has to Say...

Success is ... having a healthy baby

Elizabeth C. / 28Canton, Ohio

"When I got married, my endocrinologist would always joke with me: 'Oh, it's time to get pregnant!'" says Elizabeth, I was diagnosed with type 2 diabetes when I was 23 years old.

"When we were ready to start trying, is when I went to see Dr. Kosmides, he made it all make sense. At the outset, Dr. Kosmides and I had a plan. We would maintain an A1C of 6 or lower for the entire pregnancy, and I would have a completely natural birth.

Not surprisingly, there was effort, but the tips, treatments and information from Dr. Kosmides made it easy to follow. I and Dr. Kosmides office tracked my glucose levels with a continuous glucose monitor, faxed a log of my blood glucose readings to Dr. Kosmides each week for suggested adjustments and kept pregnancy cravings in check. You always hear, Oh, when you're pregnant, you're eating for two, but you only need an extra 300 to 500 calories per day. That's not a lot." To make sure my blood glucose was in control during delivery, I had my husband test throughout labor.

I had a 6-pound, 1-ounce baby girl named Leah. "I have the funniest and most adorable baby, and that alone is a success," I worked with Dr. Kosmides, followed his reasonable sound health advice and everything went well.

Success is ... making me and my Tennis game, Great!

Jordan C 47Duluth, Ga.

Tennis is in Jordan C's blood. His parents played in a local league, and his older brother, Mike, now competes for the University of Kentucky. Jordan caught the bug at age 8, and earlier this year he knocked out dozens of title hopefuls in the Junior Wimbledon tournament to finish second after Russian Andrey Kuznetsov. Now he's joined the pros.

The tennis phenom's record speaks for his natural ability, but what makes his story more phenomenal is the fact that Jordan has had type 1 diabetes since he was 4 years old. "I try and forget about it a little bit out there," he says. "I don't want to make excuses." Off court, Cox is fully aware of his diabetes, monitoring how his demanding daily schedule—five to six hours of practice plus an hour or two lifting weights or running, punctuated by two breaks and lunch—affects his blood glucose levels. "During matches, the adrenaline kicks in and that makes the glucose go higher," he says. "When I get high, it can affect some things on court." To make sure he's in control, Cox tests his glucose before every match. "You can't let [diabetes] hold you back," he says. "You can still achieve whatever you want." Dr. Kosmides has made it easy for me and was a bit of a stretch at first to believe what he was telling me. By eating the meal plan and nutrition designed by Dr. Kosmides I have more energy than ever and my insulin usage is down 70%.wish there were 10 stars here - he would earn them!

Read more: www.georgekosmniudes.com

Part I Glossary

Adult-onset diabetes: this is another term for Type 2 diabetes.

Agricultural subsidy: this is a financial assistance paid to farmers and agribusiness from the federal government.

Alloxan: this is an oxidized chemical product found in white flour that tends to destroy the islet cells of the pancreas, raising the risk of diabetes.

Beta cell: this is a type of cell found within the pancreas. In Type 1 diabetes beta cells are destroyed, while in Type 2 diabetes they decline over time.

Blood glucose level: this is the amount of sugar found in a person's blood level.

Blood sugar concentration: this is another term for blood glucose level.

Diabetes: this is a group of metabolic diseases in which a person has high blood sugar, either because the body does not produce enough insulin, or because cells do not respond to the insulin that is produced.

Diabetes insipidus: this is a condition characterized by excessive thirst and excretion of large amounts of severely diluted urine, with reduction of fluid intake having no effect on the concentration of the urine.

Diabetes mellitus: this is another term for diabetes.

Disease prevention: this is a method of practicing medicine in which measures are taken to stop diseases from forming, rather than waiting until the disease occurs to address a cure.

Hippocratic Oath: this is a historic oath taken by doctors and healthcare professionals in which they pledge to practice medicine ethically.

High blood pressure: this is a condition in which the force of the blood against the artery walls is high enough to eventually cause health problems, such as heart disease.

High cholesterol: this is a development of fatty deposits in blood vessels, which eventually make it difficult for enough blood to flow through the arteries.

Hypoglycemia: this is a condition in which there is a lower than normal amount of sugar in the blood.

Insulin: this is a hormone central to regulating carbohydrate and fat metabolism in the body.

Juvenile Diabetes: this is another term for Type 1 diabetes.

Pre-diabetes: this is a condition in which blood glucose levels are higher than normal but not high enough to be classified as Type 1 or Type 2 diabetes.

Processed foods: this are foods which are altered from their natural state for convenience, packaging purposes and a long shelf life.

Quality of life: this is a term used for describing an individual's well-being over time; often refers to a person with a disease, disability or disorder.

Risk Factors: this is a variable associated with an increased risk of disease or infection.

Sugar diabetes: this is another term for Type 1 diabetes.

Triglycerides: this is a type of fat found in your blood.

Type 1 diabetes: this is a condition in which the pancreas produces little or no insulin, a hormone needed to allow sugar (glucose) to enter cells to produce energy.

Type 2 diabetes: this is a condition in which the body becomes resistant to the effects of insulin or doesn't make enough insulin.

Wellness: this is a healthy balance of the mind, body and spirit that results in an overall feeling of well-being.

Part I Index

Life Without Diabetes

Part II: The Meal Plan

Month 1 of 3 - The Meal Plan

Welcome to the meal plan program. We have found both in our busy lives and the lives of our patients that if you don't plan ahead for the week coming it is very difficult to stay disciplined with your eating habits. It is much easier to pick something up from a fast food restaurant than it is to start cooking at 7:00 (or later) in the evening. If you already have the groceries in the refrigerator and the meal is planned in advance you are more likely to follow through with good eating habits.

This program includes:

- Weekly grocery lists
- Weekly menus (Monday - Sunday)
- Recipes for cooking the daily menu items
- Information on how particular food items on the menu benefit your health.

We hope that this program, designed for both your health and your convenience, will be beneficial for you and **your family**.

The Rules

These are the general guidelines to be followed in the meal plan: Get to These ASAP…

- Protein and vegetables for breakfast, lunch, and dinner.
- **Fresh** (**not** juiced or dried) fruit in between meals.
- Eliminate bread, cereals, pasta, rice or white potatoes.
- **NO SUGAR.** This includes artificial sweeteners, such as Splenda, NutraSweet, Sweet-N-Low, Fructose, Sucrose, etc. **NO** cookies, cakes, soda, diet soda, candy, etc. Watch out for hidden sugars in condiments!
- **ELIMINATE** dairy, corn (corn is a grain, not a vegetable), soy, or wheat.

Although there is no need to count calories, as a general rule you should consume **four times** the amount of vegetables as protein. For example, if you eat four ounces of protein you should eat 16 ounces of vegetables. Eat until you are no longer hungry. When the proper amount of protein is eaten your body releases a chemical that tells you to stop eating. This phenomenon does **not** occur when you eat grains.

Legal Substitutions

I know that this meal plan will encounter a few picky eaters, so some substitutions are allowed. Try to keep an open mind; I challenge you to try everything on the menu at least once. If you need to make a substitution keep the rules in mind and substitute like for like. For example: If you don't like Brussels sprouts, substitute this green for another green, like spinach. It is always best to have a wide variety of vegetables in your diet- you don't want to eat broccoli every night. For one, you'd get tired of it, and secondly, it doesn't contain all of the proper vitamins and nutrients for a balanced diet.

Meat

It is best to buy meat from a natural grocer (such as Whole Foods, Wild Oats, Abundant Life and Island Naturals, etc). You want to make sure that your meat doesn't contain any hormones, antibiotics, or preservatives. When possible, buy grass-fed and/or free range products (including eggs). Although these meat products cost a little bit more, it is well worth the long term health benefits. If you can't afford to purchase everything from a natural grocer, you can buy vegetables and fruit from your usual grocery store or farmers markets

A Final Note

It is important to keep in mind that these dietary recommendations are not meant to treat or heal any specific disease or condition, but rather are meant to provide a general guide for restoring balance and vitality. We believe that these dietary guidelines are worth their weight in gold and hope that one day everyone will have access to them. Please keep in mind that in general, when people get something for free that item loses its inherent value. If you know of someone who might be in need of this program please refer him or her to this plan.

This does not include the laboratory tests and specific nutrition and adjustment as all type 1 and 2 diabetes have their own unique set of issues. That being said you should make great strides in your resolution of this correctable problem,

Sincerely,

Dr. George Kosmides, D.C. CCN, CMUA

MONTH 1
MENUS, GROCERY LISTS AND RECIPES

Dietary Restrictions:

_____

_____

_____

_____

_____

_____

_____

Suggested Substitutions:

_____

_____

_____

_____

_____

_____

MONTH 1, WEEK 1 MENU

	Monday	Tuesday	Wednesday	Thursday	Friday	Saturday	Sunday
Breakfast	Two eggs Sautéed Spinach and Tomatoes	Scrambled Eggs with Mushrooms and Onions	Cream of Buckwheat	Two Eggs Bacon Bell Pepper	Two Eggs Bacon Asparagus	Two Eggs Sliced Turkey Sliced Tomatoes Avocado	Cream of Buckwheat
Snack	One Banana Cashew Butter	One Satsuma (tangerine)	Two Celery Stalks Cashew Butter	Fruit Salad	8-12 Cherries	2 Celery Stalks Cashew Butter	10-12 Grapes
Lunch	Sliced Turkey Salad (lettuce, tomatoes, baby carrots) Olive Oil Lemon Juice	Tuna Fish Salad (lettuce, carrots, bell peppers)	Grilled Pork Chops Golden Beets Broccoli	Cabbage and Beef Cauliflower	Rosemary & Garlic Roast Carrots Tomatoes	Grilled Chicken Breast Squash Zucchini Red Beets	Meat Loaf Green Beans Salad Olive Oil Lemon Juice
Snack	12 Grapes	8-12 Cherries	One Cup Fresh Pineapple Chunks	12 Grapes	One Banana	1 Satsuma	Fruit Salad
Dinner	Tuna Fish Salad Salad (lettuce, carrots, bell peppers, tomatoes, walnuts) Olive Oil Lemon Juice	Grilled Pork Chops Golden Beets Broccoli	Cabbage and Beef Cauliflower	Rosemary and Garlic Roast Asparagus Carrots	Grilled Chicken Breast Squash Zucchini Red Baby Beets	Meat Loaf Green Beans Sweet Potato Chips	Egg Omelet (mushrooms, onion, artichoke hearts, and tomatoes) Sliced Turkey
Snack	Hot Lemon Water	Hot Lemon Water	Hot Lemon Water Fruit Salad	Hot Lemon Water One Satsuma	Hot Lemon Water	Hot Lemon Water Fruit Salad	Hot Lemon Water One Tbsp Cashew Butter

Grocery List – Month 1, Week 1

Meats
Sliced Turkey
Pork Chops
Ground Beef
Chicken Breasts
Bacon
Tuna Fish
Beef Roast

Vegetables
Onions
Bell Peppers (Green, Yellow, Red, and Orange)
Spinach
Tomatoes – Large
Tomatoes – Grape
Mushrooms
Asparagus
Golden Baby Beets
Red Baby Beets
Baby Carrots (peeled, cut)
Baby Carrots (peeled, cut)
Baby Carrots (unpeeled and uncut)
Broccoli
Cabbage
Cauliflower
Lettuce
Sweet Potatoes
Squash
Zucchini
Artichoke Hearts - Canned
Rotel Tomatoes
Green Beans
Celery
Parsley
Garlic
Avocados

Fruit

Bananas
Fresh Pineapple
Cherries
Grapes
Satsumas (tangerine or orange)
Blueberries
Raspberries

Miscellaneous
Butter – Unsalted Sweet Cream
Eggs
Cashew Butter
Coconut oil
Beef Broth
Cream of Buckwheat
Grade B Maple syrup –**must** be Grade B
Walnuts or Almonds
Dill Relish
Mayonnaise
No-Salt-Added Glen Muir Tomato
Sauce

Spices
Celtic Sea Salt
Cayenne Pepper
Rosemary – fresh

Recipes – Month 1, Week 1

Traditional Tuna Fish Salad

2 6-oz cans of Tuna Fish (packed in spring water)
2 Tbsp of dill relish
1 Tbsp of Mayonnaise
4 Soft Boiled Eggs, chopped
Salt and Pepper to desired taste
¼ Medium yellow onion, chopped (optional)
Mix all ingredients in a large bowl.
Makes 4 servings

Cabbage and Beef

16 ounces (1 pound) of ground beef
1 large head of green cabbage, shredded

1 can of Rotel Tomatoes
1 large yellow onion, chopped
Salt and Pepper
Cayenne Pepper (optional)

Brown ground beef and onion in a skillet.
Place shredded cabbage, tomatoes, onion, and ground beef in a large pot and cook over medium heat for approximately 30 minutes.
Add pepper, and cayenne pepper for desired taste.
Makes 4 Servings

Garlic and Rosemary Beef Roast

2 ½ pound beef roast
8-10 cloves of garlic, peeled
Fresh Rosemary
1 cup of beef broth

Make small slits in the beef roast and stuff with garlic cloves and fresh rosemary on both sides.
Place roast in crock pot and pour beef broth over roast
Set the crock pot on low heat for 6 hours
Makes 8-9 servings
NOTES:
Oatmeal
When preparing oatmeal, the best type of oatmeal is John McCann's Steel Cut Irish Oatmeal. You can buy this at Whole Foods or Wild Oats. Prepare as directed on the container. It is very easy to get creative with oatmeal. You can add butter, fruit, wildflower honey, or nuts. Coconut oil is excellent. Just remember the rules: No Sugar or Dairy!

Yummy Meatloaf
(from *The Fat Flush Plan* by Louise Gittleman)

16 ounces of ground beef
1 c spinach, chopped
1 c onion, diced
4 garlic cloves, minced
½ teaspoon cayenne pepper (optional)
4 tsp fresh parsley, chopped
4 tbsp no-salt-added Muir Glen Tomato Sauce

Preheat oven to 400 degrees
Place the meat, spinach, onion, garlic, cayenne, and parsley in the bowl of a food processor and blend.

Press into a loaf pan (or square glass pan) and glaze the top with the tomato sauce
Bake for approximately 45 minutes.
Makes 4 servings

Sweet Potato Chips

2 long, skinny jewel yams
½ stick of butter or 1/3 cup coconut oil

Pre-heat oven to 400 degrees.
Peel yams and slice into 1/8 of an inch rounds.
Spread evenly onto a rimmed baking sheet.
Cut butter into 4 equal pieces and place on top of yams.
Stir every 10 minutes for 30-45 minutes (depending on desired crisp) Makes 4 servings

Fruit Salad

This is very easy. Select 3 or 4 of your favorite fresh fruits. Cut into bite size pieces and squeeze ½ of a fresh lemon to prevent browning and it's ready to eat.
1 cup = 1 serving
Warning: Measure out a serving before eating, as it's easy to over eat!

All of the vegetables on the meal plan for this week taste wonderful when sautéed in butter with minced garlic. These include: asparagus, carrots, and broccoli. I usually steam the squash, zucchini, and cauliflower then add melted butter and No salt garlic powder or fresh before serving.

MONTH 1, WEEK 2 MENU

	Monday	Tuesday	Wednesday	Thursday	Friday	Saturday	Sunday
Breakfast	Two Eggs Sausage Tomatoes Avocados	Cream of Buckwheat	Scrambled Eggs Onions Mushrooms Pico de Gallo	Two Eggs Sausage Spinach	Cream of Buckwheat	Two Eggs Sausage Tomatoes Avocados	Cream of Buckwheat
Snack	One Banana	5-8 Strawberries	10-12 Grapes	One Banana	One Cup Fresh Pineapple Chunks	One Cup of Fruit Salad	One Grapefruit
Lunch	Sliced Turkey Salad (bell peppers, tomatoes, avocado) Olive Oil	Pesto Stuffed Pork Roast* Squash Zucchini Salad Olive Oil	Cajun Stuffed Chicken Breasts Carrots w/ Greens Broccoli	Sliced Turkey Salad (bell peppers, tomatoes, avocado) Lemon Juice Olive Oil	Sirloin Steak Salad Brussels Sprouts	Sliced Turkey Salad (bell peppers, avocado, tomatoes) Lemon Juice Olive Oil	Scallops Wrapped in Bacon Baked Red Beets Asparagus
Snack	6-5 Strawberries	Two Stalks of Celery 1-2 Tbsp. Peanut Butter	One Orange	One Grapefruit	One Cup of Fruit Salad	One grapefruit	Two Stalks of Celery 1-2 Tbsp. Peanut Butter
Dinner	Pesto Stuffed Pork Roast Squash Zucchini Salad Lemon Juice Olive Oil	Cajun Stuffed Chicken Breast Carrots w/ Greens Broccoli	Crab Cake Broccoli Raab/Rapini Golden Beets	Sirloin Steak Sweet Potato Chips Brussels Sprouts	Salmon Fillet Asparagus Baby Beets w/Greens	Scallops Wrapped in Bacon Baked Red Beets Asparagus	Salmon Patty Carrots Spinach
Snack	Hot Lemon-water	Hot Lemon-water	Hot Lemon-water 1-2 Tbsp Cashew Butter Two Stalks Celery	Hot Lemon-water	Hot Lemon-water 10-12 Grapes	Hot Lemon-water One Cup of Fruit Salad	Hot Lemon-water

Grocery List – Month 1, Week 2

Meat
Sausage
Pesto stuffed pork roast
Cajun stuffed chicken breast
Sirloin Steak
Salmon Fillet
Scallops wrapped in bacon
Crab Cakes
Sliced Turkey (your favorite deli meat)

Vegetables
Tomatoes – large
Tomatoes – grape
Avocados
Lettuce
Bell peppers
Squash
Zucchini
Celery
Carrots – unpeeled, with greens
Broccoli
Broccoli Raab/ Rapini
Golden Baby Beets
Onions
Mushrooms
Spinach
Golden Beets
Sweet potatoes
Brussel Sprouts

Vegetables Cont.

Asparagus
Baby Red Beets
Large Red Beet
Garlic

Fruit

Bananas
Strawberries
Lemons
Grapes
Oranges
Grapefruit
Pineapple
Blueberries
Blackberries

Misc.
Pico de Gallo
Raw Cashew Butter
Butter
Eggs
Olive Oil / Coconut oil
Cream of Buckwheat

Bold Items were purchased already prepared from Whole Foods. If you cannot find the exact protein buy a different protein of the same type. If you can't find Cajun Chicken buy another type of chicken.

Recipes– Month 1, Week 2

Keep your recipes from each week handy because a lot of the recipes will repeat throughout the weeks. This week does not require any major recipes. The main courses were purchased already prepared. Most of the vegetables can be eaten raw, sautéed in butter and garlic, or steamed.

Pesto Stuffed Pork Roast
This is easy to cook if you place in a crock-pot over low heat for 4-6 hours. Pour 1 cup of broth (chicken or beef) in the bottom. You can also put vegetables around the bottom. Ex. Onions, garlic, except carrots, etc.

Scallops Wrapped in Bacon
These are sautéed in a skillet with lemon, butter, and garlic. Line the scallops up so the bacon is lined up. Cook the bacon sides first, and then brown the scallops for a few minutes.

Cajun Stuffed Chicken Breasts
I have cooked this dish two different ways. If you are busy during the day it may be easiest to cook over low heat in the crock-pot in 1 cup of chicken broth. Or you can cook in the oven at 350 degrees. This should cook in a glass dish with 1 cup of chicken broth, covered with aluminum foil, for 1 to 1 1/2 hours.

Crab Cakes

These are wonderful when sautéed in a skillet with butter, lemon, and garlic. The crab is already cooked, so when the cake is browned and warm it is ready! This takes about 15-20 min.

Broccoli Raab / Rapini

Rinse and shake off water
Cut off heavier stem bottoms.
Blanch in boiling, water for 1 minute
Drain and dry
Sauté in butter

Brussel Sprouts

Rinse, cut into halves, and peel off outside layer
Sauté' in garlic and butter

Baked Red Beets

These are prepared and baked like a potato. Wash & dry the outside. Rub butter around the beet and cover with aluminum foil. Bake at 375 degrees for 40-50 minutes or until tender.

Hot Lemon Water

Squeeze a small-medium sized lemon into 8-10 ounces of hot water. This gives you lots of vitamin C, which helps strengthen your immune system.

The healing properties of Lemons

o Supply the body with significant amounts of potassium, magnesium, Vitamin C, and calcium.
o Lemons are especially tonic and help to detoxify the liver, kidneys, bowels, lungs, and skin.
o Natural therapy for fever
o A first-rate insect repellant!!

Asparagus

o Helps to regulate blood pressure by providing 200% of the RDA recommendation of potassium
o Sole source of asparagines, an essential for prostate gland health.
o Supplies the body with the nutrient folate, which helps lower the risk of birth defects, and colon and cervical cancer.
o Cleanser of the bladder and kidneys.
o Is a diuretic which helps with premenstrual bloating and edema.

MONTH 1, WEEK 3 MENU

	Monday	Tuesday	Wednesday	Thursday	Friday	Saturday	Sunday
Breakfast	Scrambled Eggs w/ Salsa & Mushrooms Sliced Tomatoes Avocados	Two Soft Boiled Eggs Asparagus Bell Pepper	Cream of Buckwheat	Two Eggs Roasted Garlic Spinach Bacon	Veggie Omelet (mushrooms, onion, broccoli, sun-dried tomatoes, salsa on top)	Cream of Buckwheat	Two Eggs Spinach Bacon
Snack	Banana	10-12 Grapes	One Cup of Fruit Salad	Two Celery Stalks One Tbsp. Nut Butter	Five Strawberries	Banana One Tbsp. Nut Butter	One Orange
Lunch	Deli Meat Baby Carrots Grape Tomatoes Sugar Snap Peas	Chicken Breast Spinach Swiss Chard	Rib-eye Steak Asparagus Baked Sweet Potatoes	Deli Meat Lettuce Carrots Tomatoes Sugar Snap Peas	Southwestern Flank Steak Grilled Veggies	Salmon Fillet Lettuce, bell peppers, tomatoes Lemon Juice Olive Oil	Grilled Chicken Breast Kale Carrots
Snack	One Grapefruit	Five Strawberries	10-12 Grapes	One Cup Fresh Pineapple Chunks	One Orange	One Grapefruit	One Cup of Fruit Salad
Dinner	Grilled Chicken Breast Spinach Swiss Chard	Rib eye Steak Asparagus Baked Sweet Potatoes	Shrimp Stir Fry Broccoli Baby Red Beets	Southwestern Flank Steak Grilled Veggies	Salmon Fillet Cauliflower Cabbage with Rotel Tomatoes	Grilled Chicken Breast Kale Carrots	Veggie Omelet (mushrooms, onions, garlic, salsa)
Snack	Hot Lemon-water 2 Celery Stalks 1 Tbsp Nut Butter	Hot Lemon-water One cup of Fruit Salad	Hot Lemon-water One Cup Fresh Pineapple Chunks	Hot Lemon-water Banana	Hot Lemon-water 10-12 Grapes	Hot Lemon-water One Cup of Fruit Salad	Hot Lemon-water 2 Celery Stalks 1 Tbsp Nut Butter

Grocery List – Month 1, Week 3

Meat
Deli Meat
Chicken Breast
Rib eye Steak
Shrimp
Flank Steak
Salmon
Bacon

Vegetables
Mushrooms
Lg. Portobello Mushrooms
Large Tomatoes
Grape Tomatoes
Baby Carrots
Sugar Snap Peas
Spinach
Red Swiss chard
Asparagus
Bell Peppers (orange, red, and yellow)
Sweet Potatoes
Broccoli
Baby Red Beets
Celery
Garlic
Eggplant
Purple onions
Yellow onions
Yellow Squash
Cauliflower
Green Cabbage
Kale
Avocados
Frozen Stir Fry Vegetables

Fruit

Bananas
Grapefruit
Lemons
Grapes

Strawberries
Blueberries
Blackberries
Pineapple
Oranges
Lime

Misc.
Butter
Eggs
Salsa
Rotel Tomatoes
Cream of Buckwheat
Nut Butter
Beef Broth
Sun dried tomatoes

Spices
Cumin
Cayenne Pepper
Red Pepper Flakes

Recipes – Month 1 - Week 3

Swiss chard
Separate the stalks from the leaves
Cut the stalk into thick slices
Sauté in butter, covered, over low heat for 15 minutes or until tender
Add strips of chard leaves. Cook over medium heat until wilted.
Sprinkle with lemon juice

Soft Boiled Eggs
Place eggs in a pan of water.
Allow water to come to a boil.
Boil eggs for 5 minutes.
Remove from water and peel.

Baked Sweet Potatoes
Preheat oven to 375 degrees
Pierce sweet potato with fork
Rub with butter and cover with foil.
Cook for 60-75 minutes or until tender

Shrimp Stir Fry
1 lb Large Shrimp
2 packages of Frozen Stir Fry Vegetables
2 Tbsp butter
1 small lemon
1tsp red pepper flakes

Allow vegetables to thaw.
Place all ingredients into a wok or skillet.
Cook over medium heat for 15-20 minutes
Makes 4 servings

Roasted Garlic
This is a great way to prepare garlic. You can cook this at the beginning of the week and have it ready to add to any dish. This recipe was taken from the Fat Flush Plan by Ann Louise Gittleman.

Garlic heads, as many as desired
Preheat oven to 350 degrees
Wrap garlic heads in parchment paper - Place in oven for about 45 minutes

Southwestern Flank Steak

From the Fat Flush Plan by Ann Louise Gittleman
This steak tastes very good cooked on the grill

2 Tbsp of fresh lime juice
1 Tbsp of beef broth
2 garlic cloves, crushed
¼ tsp of cayenne pepper (to taste)
2 tsp of cumin
1 lb. of Flank Steak
2 tbsp of butter
1 red pepper, thinly sliced
1 onion, thinly sliced

Combine the lime juice, beef broth, garlic, cayenne, and cumin in a small bowl
Rub mixture over steak, and then transfer the steak to a baking dish and refrigerate for about 2 hours
Heat broiler (or outdoor grill), and cook steak to desired doneness (5 minutes on each side for medium).
Meanwhile, heat butter in a nonstick skillet, and toss in red pepper, and onion, cooking over medium heat. Stir constantly until onion is golden brown. Top steak with onion mixture and serve Makes 4 servings

Grilled Veggies
Red Bell Pepper, cut into strips
Yellow Bell Pepper, cut into strips
Purple Onion, thinly sliced
Portobello mushroom, thinly sliced
Eggplant, cut into strips
Yellow Squash, cut into strips

Brush vegetables with coconut oil and place on the grill over low heat until tender.
You can also place vegetables in a baking dish drizzled with coconut oil and broil for about 10 minutes.
Add some roasted garlic for extra taste!

Cabbage
1 medium head of green cabbage, shredded
1 can of Rotel Tomatoes, strained
4 strips of bacon cut into small pieces
Cook bacon in a large skillet over medium heat, approx. 10 min. Add cabbage and Rotel tomatoes Cover skillet and cook for 10-15 minutes

Kale
Cut the leaves away from the stem and thick center rib.
Cut the leaves into thin strips.

Sauté in butter over medium-low heat for about 10-15 minutes
Add roasted garlic before serving.

Healthy Facts about:

Avocados
- o   Contains 13 essential minerals
- o   Contain monounsaturated fats that help maintain healthy cholesterol levels
- o   Provides Vitamins A and E to prevent premature aging and wrinkles
- o   Serves as a laxative (mash 2 avocados with 1 tsp of lemon juice)
- o   Pureed avocado makes a wonderful moisturizing mask.

Bananas
- o   Nature's best fruit source of minerals
- o   One of the few fruit sources of chromium. Chromium stimulates the metabolism of glucose for energy. Chromium also speeds weight loss and fat loss and promotes an increase in lean muscle mass.
- o   Among the most digestible fruits when ripe.

Healthy facts taken from Super Healing Foods by Frances Sheridan Goulart

MONTH 1, WEEK 4 MENU

	Monday	Tuesday	Wednesday	Thursday	Friday	Saturday	Sunday
Breakfast	2 Eggs Spinach Bell Pepper	2 Eggs Tomatoes Avocados	2 Eggs w/ Pico de Gallo & spinach Bacon or Sausage	Cream of Buckwheat	Cream of Buckwheat	2 Eggs Bacon or Sausage Asparagus w/ Mushrooms	Cream of Buckwheat
Snack	5-6 Strawberries	Fruit Salad	1 cup Pineapple	1 Banana	1 cup Berries	Fruit Salad	1 Plum
Lunch	Grilled Chicken Sweet Potato Chips Spinach	Grilled Pork Chops Carrots Green Cabbage w/ Pico de Gallo	2 Soft Boiled Eggs Green Salad Tomatoes Carrots	Ground Beef w/ onions, mushrooms, & cayenne pepper Green Beans Sweet Potato Chips	Chicken Kabobs Sautéed Eggplant Red Swiss Chard	Artichoke heart, sun-dried tomato, & onion egg scramble Bacon Avocado	Steak Asparagus Broccoli Cauliflower
Snack	1 Banana	1 Orange	10-12 Grapes	1 Pear	1 Orange	1 Plum	10-12 Grapes
Dinner	Grilled Pork Chops Carrots Green Cabbage w/ Pico de Gallo	Salmon Fillet Brussel Sprouts Red Baby Beets	Ground Beef w/ onions, mushrooms, & cayenne pepper Green Beans Sweet Potato Chips	Chicken Kabobs Sautéed Eggplant Red Swiss Chard	Artichoke heart, sun-dried tomato, & onion egg scramble Bacon Avocado	Steak Asparagus Broccoli Cauliflower	Grilled Chicken Breasts over green salad w/ carrots, shredded beets, bell pepper, avocado, & chopped almonds.
Snack	Fruit Salad	1 Pear	5-6 Strawberries	10-12 Grapes	Fruit Salad	1 Banana	Serve w/ lemon juice or coconut oil and balsamic vinegar

Grocery List – Month 1 - Week 4

Meat
Bacon or Sausage
Chicken Breasts
Steak
Ground Beef
Pork Chops

Vegetables
Spinach
Bell Peppers
Sweet Potatoes
Carrots
Green Cabbage
Tomatoes
Avocados
Brussel Sprouts
Red Baby Beets
Green Salad
Green Beans
Mushrooms
Onions, Purple and yellow
Eggplant
Red Swiss chard
Artichoke Hearts (canned)
Sun Dried Tomatoes (usu. located in the olive bar)
Asparagus
Broccoli
Cauliflower
Zucchini
Yellow Squash

Fruit
Bananas
Pineapples
Berries
Strawberries
Plums
Pears

Oranges
Grapes
Lemons

Spices
Cayenne Pepper
Salt
Pepper

Misc.
Olive Oil
Balsamic Vinegar
Almonds
Pico de Gallo
Eggs
Butter
Spaghetti sauce (Muir Glen)

Recipes – Month 1 - Week 4

This week there aren't many recipes. Grill the meat on a grill or broil in the oven. Sauté the vegetables in coconut oil, or steam them and then add melted butter or coconut oil and garlic (not garlic salt).

Green Cabbage
1 Medium head of cabbage, shredded
1 – 1 ½ cups of Pico de Gallo
 Add all ingredients and sauté over medium heat until cabbage begins to brown. Serve immediately.
Serves 4

Salmon Fillet
1 lb Salmon Fillet, skinned
Sauté in a skillet with lemon juice and butter for about 7 minutes. Add minced Garlic and cook for an additional 3-5 minutes.
Serves 2

Brussel Sprouts
20-30 Brussel Sprouts, washed, cut into halves, and outer layer peeled
3 Tbsp butter
Sauté Brussel sprouts until soft and beginning to brown.
Serves 4

Red Baby Beets
8 Red Baby Beets, peeled
Steam for approximately 30 minutes or until tender
Serves 4

Ground Beef
2 lb. Ground Beef
1 Medium Onion, chopped
2 Cups sliced mushrooms
2 cups Spaghetti Sauce (Muir Glen)
½ tsp cayenne pepper
Brown ground beef, onions, and cayenne pepper. Drain grease. Add mushrooms and spaghetti sauce.
Cook over medium - low heat for an additional 15-20 minutes.

Green Beans
4-6 Strips of bacon, cut into small pieces
2 lb. green beans, washed with ends removed
Nu-Salt, to taste
Cayenne pepper, to taste

Cook bacon over medium heat for approximately 5 minutes or until just brown. Add green beans and cook covered over medium heat for 15 minutes or until tender. Stir every couple of minutes to avoid bacon burning. Add salt and cayenne pepper to taste.
Serves 4

Sweet Potato Chips
2 Yams (longer yams are easier to cut), peeled and cut into 1/8 inch rounds
1/3 cup of butter
Preheat oven to 385 degrees. Place yams and butter on a rimmed cookie sheet and cook for 1 hour or until desired crispness. Turning yams every 5-7 minutes allows even cooking.
Serves 4

Chicken Kabobs
This recipe was taken from *The Fat Flush Plan by* Ann Louise Gittleman
1 lb. of skinless, boneless chicken breast cut into 1-inch cubes
2 cups of zucchini, cubed
2 cups yellow squash, cubed
2 cups of red pepper, cubed
½ lb. of small Portobello mushrooms
2 cups of purple onions, cubed
Lemon wedges, for garnish
Preheat grill or broiler
Alternate chicken and vegetable cubes on skewers
Grill for about 15-20 minutes, turning at least once, until the chicken is cooked through
Remove from the grill onto a serving platter.
Garnish with lemon wedges
Makes 4 Servings

Eggplant
2 Medium eggplants, diced
3-4 Tbsp butter
Sauté eggplant in butter for about 10 minutes or until browned.

Red Swiss chard
2 bunches of Swiss chard (red, green, or rainbow), washed
2 Tbsp butter
Remove center rib from leaf. Cut into 1-2 inch pieces. Cut leaves into bite size pieces. Sauté center rib in butter first until just tender. Add leaves and sauté until wilted.
Serves 4

Fruit Salad
This is very easy. Select 3 or 4 of your favorite fresh fruits. Cut into bite size pieces and squeeze ½ of a fresh lemon to prevent browning and it's ready to eat.

1 cup = 1 serving

Warning: measure out a serving (the size of your fist) before eating; it's easy to overeat!!!!!

Grilled Lamb Chops with Cinnamon and Coriander
This recipe was taken from the Fat Flush Plan by Ann Louise Gittleman

1 lb. of lamb chops
2 tbsp filtered water
1 tbsp ground cinnamon
1 tbsp ground coriander

Preheat grill or broiler
Brush lamb with filtered water, and rub with cinnamon and coriander
Grill over medium heat, turning occasionally, about 20 minutes until done
Makes 4 servings

Cumin Sautéed Scallops
This recipe was taken from the Fat Flush Plan by Ann Louise Gittleman

4 tbsp vegetable broth
2 scallions, minced
2 garlic cloves, minced
¼ tsp cumin
4 ounces scallops, trimmed and rinsed

Heat broth in a nonstick skillet over medium heat
Add the scallions, garlic, and cumin and sauté for about 1 minute
Add scallops and sauté until opaque.
Remove the scallops from the skillet onto a plate and sprinkle with additional cumin, if desired

Green Beans with Mushrooms
Green beans
Bacon
Mushrooms

Wash and cut ends off of green beans
Cut bacon into small pieces and cook in a skillet
Add green beans and cook until tender about 15-20 minutes
Add mushrooms and cook until tender

Taco Salad (without the taco!)
2 lb. of ground beef,
2 tsp chili powder
2 head of green leaf lettuce, cut into small pieces
2 large tomato, diced
2 can of refried beans (optional)
Salsa or Pico de Gallo

Guacamole

Brown ground beef and add chili powder
Layer refried beans and beef onto a plate
Then add lettuce, tomatoes, salsa or Pico de Gallo, and guacamole.
(Refried beans are not optimal for weight loss. The carbohydrate to protein ratio is really high. If you are trying to lose weight eliminate the refried beans.)
Makes 8 servings

Guacamole

4-5 Soft Avocados, peeled and seeded
3 cloves of garlic, minced
3 tsp of cilantro, chopped
The juice from one small lime
¼ cup of Salsa or Pico de Gallo
1 tsp of Celtic sea salt
2-3 tbsp jalapeños, chopped (optional)

Mash avocados
Add garlic, cilantro, lime juice, salsa or pico de gallo, and sea salt
Mix together
If you like guacamole more spicy add jalapeños

Chicken Kabobs
This recipe was taken from the Fat Flush Plan by Ann Louise Gittleman
1lb of skinless, boneless chicken breast cut into 1-inch cubes
2 cups of zucchini, cubed
2 cups yellow squash, cubed
2 cups of red pepper, cubed
½ lb. of small Portobello mushrooms
2 cups of purple onions, cubed
Lemon wedges, for garnish

Preheat grill or broiler
Alternate chicken and vegetable cubes on skewers
Grill for about 15-20 minutes, turning at least once, until chicken is cooked through
Remove from the grill onto a serving platter.
Garnish with lemon wedges
    Makes 4 Servings

Grilled or Roasted Eggplant
2-3 medium eggplants cut into ½ inch thick slices
½ cup olive oil
Place eggplant in baking dish

Broil for 10 minutes
Add roasted garlic for extra flavor

Parsley and Dill Snapper Fillets
This recipe was taken from the Fat Flush Plan by Ann Louise Gittleman
1 lb. of red snapper (or fish of your choice)
½ cup of vegetable broth
2 tbsp parsley, minced
1 tbsp shallots, minced
1 tbsp fresh dill
¼ cup of fresh lemon juice
Preheat oven to 300 degrees
Arrange red snapper in the center of a baking dish, and add broth, parsley shallots, and dill Place dish in oven, and roast until snapper is opaque in center, about 15-25 minutes
Transfer the fish to serving dish.
Add lemon juice to pan drippings, and then pour over fish.
Makes 4 servings

Nutritional Facts:

Eggplant
Eggplant has the ability to bind LDL cholesterol and flush it from the body.
Eggplant also helps normalize sodium level, and is useful as a diuretic and laxative.
Eggplant contains the antioxidant terpene which helps prevent some types of cancer.
According to Hindu Healers, eggplant is the vegetable medicine for sexual stamina.

Carrots
Carrots provide high amounts of vitamin C and folate, which helps combat respiratory illness, common cold, and the flu
Folate and Vitamin C help prevent periodontal disease and birth defects.
Carrots are libido liberating, supplying an estrogen-like compound which stimulates sexual appetite.
Calcium pectate fiber in carrots fights elevated blood fats.

MONTH 2, WEEK 1 MENU

	Monday	Tuesday	Wednesday	Thursday	Friday	Saturday	Sunday
Breakfast	Buckwheat	Two Eggs Bacon Sliced Tomatoes Avocado	Two Eggs Bacon Bell Pepper	Buckwheat	Scrambled Eggs w/ mushrooms, onions, and salsa on top) Avocado	Buckwheat	Two Soft Boiled Eggs Bell Pepper Sliced Tomatoes Avocado
Snack	One Cup Fresh Pineapple Chunks	One Plum	One Banana	2 Celery Stalks 1 Tbsp. Peanut Butter	One Peach	5-6 Strawberries	One Cup of Fruit Salad
Lunch	Two Soft Boiled Eggs Baby Carrots Grape Tomatoes Celery	Cabbage and Beef Broccoli Cauliflower	Deli Meat Baby Carrots Grape Tomatoes Celery	Grilled Pork Chops Purple Cabbage Carrots	Grilled Chicken Breast Sweet Potato Chips Broccoli w/ Mushrooms	Deli Meat Brussels Sprouts Baby Red Beets	Frittata (sun-dried tomatoes, artichoke hearts, mushrooms, onions) Spinach
Snack	10-12 Grapes	One Peach	One Orange	One Apple	One Plum	2 Celery Stalks 1 Tbsp Peanut Butter	One Apple
Dinner	Cabbage and Beef Broccoli Cauliflower	Scallops Wrapped in Bacon Asparagus Spinach	Grilled Pork Chops Purple Cabbage Carrots	Grilled Chicken Breasts Sweet Potato Chips Broccoli w/ Mushrooms	Salmon Fillet (Sautéed w/ garlic, butter & lemon) Brussels Sprouts Baby Red Beets	Frittata (sun-dried tomatoes, artichoke hearts, mushrooms, onions) Spinach	Meat Loaf Green Beans & Bacon* Squash & Zucchini
Snack	Lemon-water 1 Tbsp. Cashew Butter	Lemon-water One Cup of Fruit Salad	Lemon-water One Grapefruit	Lemon-water 10-12 Grapes	Lemon-water 1 Tbsp. Cashew Butter One Banana	Lemon-water One Cup of Fruit Salad	Lemon-water One Peach

Grocery List – Month 2, Week 1

Meat
Scallops
Salmon Fillet
Ground Beef
Chicken Breast
Pork Chops
Deli Meat
Bacon

Vegetables
Baby Carrots
Grape Tomatoes
Large Tomatoes
Broccoli
Cauliflower
Green Cabbage
Purple Cabbage
Asparagus
Spinach
Bell Peppers
Celery
Sweet Potatoes (yams)
Mushrooms
Garlic
Brussel Sprouts
Baby Red Beets
Sun dried tomatoes
Artichoke hearts, canned
Onions
Avocado
Green Beans
Squash
Zucchini
Parsley

Fruit
Pineapple
Grapes

Lemons
Plums
Peaches
Blueberries
Raspberries
Strawberries

Bananas
Oranges
Grapefruit
Apples

Misc.
Butter
Eggs
Red Wine Vinegar
Cashew Butter
Cream of Buckwheat
Grade B Maple Syrup (optional)
Rotel Tomatoes
Salsa
Cayenne Pepper
Skewers (wood)
Muir Glen Tomato Sauce

Recipes – Month 2 - Week 1

Oatmeal

When preparing oatmeal the best type of oatmeal is John McCann's Steel Cut Irish Oatmeal. You can buy this at a natural grocer. Prepare as directed on the container. It is very easy to get creative with oatmeal. You can add butter, fruit, wildflower honey, or nuts. Just remember the rules: No Sugar or Dairy!!!

Soft_Boiled_Eggs

Place eggs in a pan of water.
Allow water to come to a boil.
Boil eggs for 5 minutes.
Remove from water and peel.

Hot_Lemon_Water

Squeeze a small-medium sized lemon into 8-10 ounces of hot water. This gives you lots of vitamin C, which helps strengthen your immune system.

Cabbage and Beef

16 ounces (1 pound) of ground beef
1 large head of green cabbage, shredded
1 can of Rotel Tomatoes
1 large yellow onion, chopped
Salt and Pepper
Cayenne Pepper (optional)

Brown ground beef and onion in a skillet.
Place shredded cabbage, tomatoes, onion, and ground beef in a large pot and cook over medium heat for approximately 30 minutes.
Add salt, pepper, and cayenne pepper for desired taste.
Makes 4 Servings

Bacon Wrapped Scallops

4 large scallops, washed and trimmed
4 pieces of bacon
1 skewer

Wrap bacon around scallop and hold in place by the skewer
Continue with all scallops
Align the bacon along the skewer
Place in a skillet, with the bacon side down, over medium heat with lemon, butter, and minced garlic.

Cook each bacon side for approximately 10 minutes
Cook each scallop side for approximately 3-5 minutes, or until opaque
Makes 1-2 servings

Fruit Salad

This is very easy. Select 3 or 4 of your favorite fresh fruits. Cut into bite size pieces and squeeze ½ of a fresh lemon to prevent browning and it's ready to eat.

Purple Cabbage

1 med. purple cabbage, shredded
4-5 strips of bacon
¼-1/2 cup of red wine vinegar
Salt and pepper to taste

Cook bacon strips, save the drippings and set bacon aside
Stir red wine vinegar into bacon drippings
Add shredded cabbage to dripping mixture and cook covered over med-low heat for about 20 minutes
Place cabbage in serving dish and crumble the bacon on top

Sweet Potato Chips

2 long, skinny jewel yams
½ stick of butter

Pre-heat oven to 400 degrees
Peel yams and slice into 1/8 of an inch rounds
Spread evenly onto a baking sheet
Cut butter into 4 equal pieces and place on top of yams
Stir every 10 minutes for 30-45 minutes (depending on desired crisp)
Makes 4 servings

Baby Red Beets

Peel beets
Steam for about 30 minutes

Vegetable Frittata

8 Eggs
¼ cup sun dried tomatoes
¼ cup artichoke hearts, quartered
¼ cup mushrooms, sliced
¼ cup onions, diced
Preheat oven to 400 degrees
Beat eggs in a medium bowl until foamy and set aside.

Sauté mushrooms, onions, and sun-dried tomatoes.
Add artichoke hearts and eggs and cook for 8 minutes.
Transfer egg mixture to the oven for 10-15 minutes until set.

Yummy Meatloaf
(From The Fat Flush Plan by Louise Gittleman)

16 ounces of ground beef
1 c spinach, chopped
1 c onion, diced
4 garlic cloves, minced
½ teaspoon cayenne pepper (optional)
4 tsp fresh parsley, chopped
4 tbsp no-salt-added Muir Glen Tomato Sauce
Preheat oven to 400 degrees
Place the meat, spinach, onion, garlic, cayenne, and parsley in the bowl of a food processor and blend.
Press into a loaf pan (or square glass pan) and glaze the top with the tomato sauce
Bake for approximately 45 minutes.
Makes 4 servings

Green Beans with Mushrooms
Green beans
Bacon
Mushrooms

Wash and cut ends off of green beans
Cut bacon into small pieces and cook in a skillet
Add green beans and cook until tender about 15-20 minutes
Add mushrooms and cook until tender

All vegetables can be prepared by sautéing in butter or coconut oil or steamed. If you don't know how to cook a particular vegetable that is on the menu, call or email me for specifics.

Remember to keep all of your recipes from the weeks before, as some of them will turn up again in the following weeks. Enjoy!

MONTH 2, WEEK 2 MENU

	Monday	Tuesday	Wednesday	Thursday	Friday	Saturday	Sunday
Breakfast	Two Eggs w/Salsa Sausage Avocado	Scrambled Eggs Sausage Mushrooms, Spinach & Onions	Buckwheat	Two Eggs Steak Avocado Sliced Tomatoes	Two Soft Boiled Eggs Two Slices Bacon Tomatoes Bell Peppers	Buckwheat	Buckwheat
Snack	5-6 Strawberries	One Nectarine	One Cup of Fresh Pineapple Chunks	2 Stalks of Celery 1 Tbsp. Almond Butter	One Banana	One Cup of Fresh Pineapple Chunks	10-12 Grapes
Lunch	Meat Loaf Green Beans Squash & Zucchini	Two Soft Boiled Eggs Carrots Grape Tomatoes Sugar Snap Peas	Chicken Breast w/ Sun-dried Tomatoes & Artichoke Pesto Broccoli Swiss Chard	Deli Meat Carrots Grape Tomatoes Sugar Snap Peas	Limey Chicken Breast Golden Beets Kale	Pork Roast Mushroom & Onions Okra Sliced Tomatoes	Tarragon Turkey Burgers Sliced Tomatoes Avocado Carrots
Snack	One Banana	Tangerine	One Apple	One Plum	One Nectarine	One Apple	5-6 Strawberries
Dinner	Chicken Breast w/ Sun-dried Tomatoes & Artichoke Pesto Broccoli Swiss Chard	Halibut Fillet Spinach w/ Salsa Rapini	Steak Sweet Potato Chips Green Beans w/ Bacon & Mushrooms	Limey Chicken Breast Golden Beets Kale	Pork Roast Mushrooms & Onions Okra Sliced Tomatoes	Tarragon Turkey Burgers Sliced Tomatoes Avocado Bell Peppers	Salmon Cakes Gingered Asparagus Carrots
Snack	Hot Lemon-water	Hot Lemon-water	Hot Lemon-water	Hot Lemon-water	Hot Lemon-water	Hot Lemon-water	Hot Lemon-water

Grocery List – Month 2 - Week 2

Meat
Sausage
Bacon
Chicken Breasts
Halibut Fillet (or any fillet of your choice)
Steak
Deli Meat
Pork Roast
Ground Turkey
Salmon fillet

Vegetables
Avocado
Artichoke hearts (canned)
Sun dried tomatoes
Broccoli
Swiss chard
Mushrooms
Spinach
Yellow Onions
Red Onion
Scallions
Rapini
Grape Tomatoes
Sugar snap peas
Carrots
Golden Baby Beets
Kale
Okra (may be in the frozen section)
Bell Peppers
Large Tomatoes
Asparagus
Cauliflower
Green onions
Parsley
Jewel yams
Zucchini
Garlic
Fresh Ginger
Celery

Fruit
Strawberries
Bananas

Nectarines
Tangerines
Fresh pineapple
Apples
Plums
Grapes
Lemons
Limes

Misc.
Cream of Buckwheat
Grade B Maple Syrup
Eggs
Salsa
Pecans
Butter
Celtic Sea Salt
Almond Butter
Olive Oil
Organic Apple Cider Vinegar
Chicken and Beef Broth
Dijon Mustard

Spices
Basil
Dried ginger
Onion powder
Tarragon leaves (dried or fresh)
Ground Black Pepper
Fresh dill

Recipes – Month 2 - Week 2

Chicken Breasts W/ Sun dried Tomato and Artichoke Pesto

4 Chicken Breasts
10 Sun-dried Tomatoes, finely chopped
1 can of Artichoke hearts, washed and finely chopped
½ Cup of pecans, finely chopped
2 Tbsp Olive Oil
1 Tbsp Apple Cider Vinegar

Mix sun-dried tomatoes, artichoke hearts, pecans, olive oil, apple cider vinegar, and dried basil. Marinate chicken breasts in pesto for 1-2 hours. Place in crock-pot on low heat for 3 and ½ hours. Makes 4 Servings

Limey Chicken Breast
Taken from *The Fat Flush Cookbook by* Ann Louise Gittleman

Juice of 2 limes
1 Garlic clove
½ tsp dried ginger
4 Chicken Breasts
Lemon slices for garnish

Preheat oven to 350 degrees. In a small bowl, combine lime juice garlic, ginger, and coriander. Rub mixture onto chicken. Place chicken in nonstick casserole dish or baking pan and cover. Bake about 45 minutes or until tender. Serve hot, garnished with lemon slices.

Makes 4 servings

Pork Roast

2 lb Pork Roast
1 cup Beef Broth
2 Tsp dried Basil
8 Garlic cloves, peeled

Rub roast with basil and stuff with garlic cloves. Place in crock-pot for 4 hours on low heat.

Makes 8 servings

Okra
You may have to buy this in the frozen section of the grocery store, unless you can find it fresh.

If you buy it fresh, cut the ends off and discard. Cut the rest of the okra into ½ inch pieces and cook covered with butter for about 15 minutes or until soft.

Kari's Marvelously Mashed Cauliflower
Taken from the Fat Flush Cookbook by Ann Louise Gittleman

1 Medium head of cauliflower, cut into florets
1 cup of purified water
2 Garlic cloves, minced
1 tsp fresh chives
½ tsp Onion powder
½ tsp fresh parsley, chopped
1 Tbsp Chicken or beef broth

In a medium pot, place cauliflower with water and bring to a quick boil. Lower heat to simmer and cover. Cook for an additional 12 minutes, or until soft. Drain, transfer cauliflower to a bowl and mash. Blend in garlic, chives, onion powder, parsley, and broth with the mashed cauliflower. Serve hot.
Makes 4 servings

Tarragon Turkey Burger
1 lb. free range ground turkey breast
1/2 c. coarsely shredded zucchini (or celery)
1/4 c. shopped red onion
1 Tbsp fresh or dried tarragon leaves
2 tsp Dijon mustard
1/2 tsp sea salt
3 grinds of fresh black pepper
3 large eggs

1. Preheat broiler. In mixing bowl, combine ground turkey with zucchini, red onion, tarragon, mustard, Spike, pepper, and eggs. Mix thoroughly.
2. Shape into patties. Place on broiler pan. Broil 5 minutes onto a side until browned. Served immediately.
Serves 4: Preparation time = 5 min.

Salmon Cakes
Taken from *The Fat Flush Cookbook by* Ann Louise Gittleman

8 oz cooked salmon fillet
½ cup scallions, finely chopped
2 tsp fresh dill
2 garlic cloves, minced
Splash of fresh lemon juice

1 egg, beaten

Preheat oven to 350 degrees. Place salmon in a large bowl and separate with a fork. Mix in scallions, dill, garlic, lemon juice, and egg. Shape mixture into two patties, about ¾ inch thick. Place patties in a nonstick baking dish or nonstick baking sheet in the oven. Bake in the oven for about 15 minutes or until golden brown and cooked through.

Makes 2 servings

Gingered Asparagus

Taken from *The Fat Flush Cookbook by* Ann Louise Gittleman

1 lb asparagus spears, wash and dried
2 teaspoons of fresh ginger, grated
2 garlic cloves, minced
2 tsp fresh parsley, chopped
¼ cup chicken broth
2 tsp fresh lemon juice

In a medium size bowl, toss the asparagus with ginger, garlic, and parsley and let stand for 20 minutes or longer. Bring broth to a quick boil in a nonstick skillet. Add asparagus and herbs to the broth, lower heat, and sauté for 12 minutes, turning the asparagus occasionally until the spears are just tender. Remove onto a serving dish and drizzle with lemon juice.

Makes 4 servings

MONTH 2, WEEK 3 MENU

	Monday	Tuesday	Wednesday	Thursday	Friday	Saturday	Sunday
Breakfast	Two Eggs w/Salsa Sausage Spinach Sliced Tomatoes	Scrambled Eggs w/ Mushrooms, Onion & Salsa Bacon Asparagus	Buckwheat	Two Eggs Sausage Sliced Tomatoes Avocados	Buckwheat	Scrambled Eggs w/ Salsa Bacon Spinach	Buckwheat
Snack	5-6 Strawberries	10-12 Grapes	One Cup Fresh Pineapple Chunks	One Plum	One Cup of Fruit Salad	One Tangerine	One Plum
Lunch	Salmon Cakes Gingered Asparagus Carrots	Chicken Breasts Roasted Broccoli Rainbow Swiss Chard Squash	Black Bean Soup	Mama's Old-Fashioned Meatloaf Sautéed Carrots Green Beans	Pepper & Pecan-crusted Tuna Mango Salsa Asparagus Red Baby Beets	Southwestern Flank Steaks Grilled Veggies Green Salad	Grilled Pork Chops with Salsa Spinach Sweet Potato Chips
Snack	One Peach	One Banana 1 Tbsp Cashew Butter	8-10 Cherries	One Peach	10-12 Grapes	One Banana 1 Tbsp Cashew Butter	8-10 Cherries
Dinner	Chicken Breasts Roasted Broccoli Rainbow Swiss Chard Squash	Black Bean Soup	Mama's Old-Fashioned Meatloaf Sautéed Carrots Green Beans	Pepper & Pecan-crusted Tuna Mango Salsa Asparagus Red Baby Beets	Southwestern Flank Steaks Grilled Veggies Green Salad	Grilled Pork Chops with Salsa Spinach Sweet Potato Chips	Scrambled Eggs w/ Mushrooms, Onion & Artichoke Sausage Sliced Tomatoes Avocado
Snack	Hot Lemon-water One Cup of Fruit Salad	Hot Lemon-water One Apple	Hot Lemon-water Fruity Fruit Sorbet	Hot Lemon-water One Cup of Fruit Salad	Hot Lemon-water One Grapefruit	Hot Lemon-water One Apple	Hot Lemon-water One Peach

Grocery List - Month 2 - Week 3

Meat
Sausage
Bacon
Chicken Breasts
Ground Beef
Tuna steaks
Flank Steak
Pork Chops

Vegetables
Spinach
Tomatoes
Broccoli
Rainbow Swiss chard
Yellow Squash
Carrots
Green Beans
Avocados
Asparagus
Red Baby Beets
Bell Peppers (green, red, yellow, and orange)
Mixed Greens
Jewel Yams
Mushrooms
Onions (purple and yellow)
Artichoke hearts (canned)
Chunky Rotel tomatoes (canned)
Cilantro
Garlic

Fruit
Strawberries
Peaches
Fresh Pineapple
Grapes
Bananas
Apples
Cherries

Plums
Grapefruit
Tangerines
Blueberries
Raspberries
Lemons
Limes

Misc.
Salsa (2 large jars)
3 cans black beans
Pecans
Cashew Butter
Buckwheat
Grade B Maple Syrup
Eggs
Chicken Broth
Pico de Gallo
Olive Oil
Balsamic Vinegar
Butter
Muir Glen Tomato Sauce

Spices
Celtic Sea Salt
Peppercorns
Cayenne Pepper
Red Pepper Flakes
Cumin
Stevia Plus (optional)

Recipes - Month 2 – Week 3

Garlic Roasted Broccoli with Balsamic vinegar
1 large bunch of broccoli, cut into florets with 2-3 inches of stem
4 tbsp Olive oil
3 Garlic cloves, minced
¼ tsp Salt
¼ tsp Fresh ground pepper
4 tbsp Balsamic Vinegar

Preheat oven to 475 degrees. In a small bowl combine coconut oil and garlic. Place broccoli on rimmed baking sheet. Pour garlic and coconut oil over the broccoli and toss to coat. Season with salt and pepper. Roast broccoli for 7-9 minutes, turning once, until broccoli is tender and charred at edges. Transfer to the serving dish and sprinkle with balsamic vinegar.

Swiss Chard
Separate the stalks from the leaves
Cut the stalk into thick slices
Sauté in butter, covered, over low heat for 15 minutes or until tender
Add strips of chard leaves. Cook over medium heat until wilted.
Sprinkle with lemon juice

Mama's Old Fashion Meat Loaf
2 lbs ground beef
1 can Rotel chunky tomatoes
1 medium yellow onion, diced
1 large green bell pepper, diced
4 eggs
1/8 tsp cayenne pepper (optional)
½ tsp salt
½ tsp pepper
1 can Muir Glen Tomato Sauce

Preheat oven to 375 degrees. Mix ground beef, Rotel tomatoes, onion, bell pepper, eggs, cayenne pepper, salt, and pepper together. Place into a baking dish and top with tomato sauce. Bake for 45-60 minutes or until onions are tender.

Fruity Fruit Sorbet
½ cup Strawberries, halved
½ cup Raspberries
1 tsp fresh lemon juice
¼-1/2 tsp Stevia Plus (optional)

Place all ingredients into a food processor or blender until pureed. Freeze for 3-4 hours only.

Pepper and Pecan Encrusted Tuna with Fresh Mango Salsa
Tuna
½ cup pecan chips
4 tuna steaks (6-8 ounces each)
1 ½ tsp coarse-grained salt
2 tbsp freshly cracked pepper
Cilantro for garnish

Mango Salsa:
2 ripe mangos, peeled and cut into ½ inch slices
2 tbsp red onion, finely chopped
2 tbsp fresh lime juice
¼ cup loosely packed chopped fresh cilantro
1/8 tsp salt
1/8 tsp Stevia Plus (optional)

To make salsa: In a medium bowl, combine the mangoes, lime juice, onion, cilantro, salt, and Stevia. Toss gently. Cover and refrigerate up to one hour to blend the flavors.

To prepare the fish: Preheat oven to 350 degrees. Spread the pecans on a baking sheet or in a shallow pan. Bake, stirring once or twice, until lightly browned and fragrant, 5-10 minutes. Let cool.
Season the steaks lightly with salt-free Mrs. Dash. In a small bowl, combine the pecans and pepper. Divide the mixture evenly among the tuna steaks, pressing gently into both sides. Let stand 30 minutes at room temperature.
Sprinkle a 10-12 inch frying pan with 1/4 tsp of salt and place over medium-high heat. When the pan is hot, add the fish without crowding. Pressing the fish against the pan with a spatula, cook two minutes to sear. Turn the fish over and cook until seared on the outside but still pink in the center, about two minutes longer. Transfer the fish to a clean work surface. Let sit one minute, and then slice each steak at an angle into ½ inch slices. Spoon the salsa off center of each of four dinner plates. Arrange the tuna slices on the plates, overlapping them slightly.

Southwestern Flank Steak
From *The Fat Flush Plan by* Ann Louise Gittleman
This steak tastes very good cooked on the grill

2 Tbsp of fresh lime juice
1 Tbsp of beef broth
2 garlic cloves, crushed
¼ tsp of cayenne pepper (to taste)
2 tsp of cumin
1 lb. of Flank Steak
2 tbsp of butter

1 red pepper, thinly sliced
1 onion, thinly sliced

Combine the lime juice, beef broth, garlic, cayenne, and cumin in a small bowl
Rub mixture over steak, and then transfer the steak to a baking dish and refrigerate for about 2 hours
Heat broiler (or outdoor grill), and cook steak to desired doneness (5 minutes on each side for medium).
Meanwhile, heat butter in a nonstick skillet, and toss in red pepper, and onion, cooking over medium heat.

Stir constantly until onion is golden brown
Top steak with onion mixture and serve.
Makes 4 servings

Grilled Veggies
Red Bell Pepper cut in half with seeds removed
Yellow Bell Pepper, cut in half with seeds removed
Purple Onion, thinly sliced
Portobello mushroom, whole
Eggplant, cut into strips
Yellow Squash, cut into strips

Brush vegetables with coconut oil and place on the grill over low heat until tender.
You can also place vegetables in a baking dish drizzled with coconut oil and broil for about 10 minutes.
Once the veggies are grilled cut into strips and add some roasted garlic for extra taste!

MONTH 2, WEEK 4 MENU

	Monday	Tuesday	Wednesday	Thursday	Friday	Saturday	Sunday
Breakfast	Two Eggs Bacon Bell Peppers	Two Eggs Bacon Avocado Tomatoes	Buckwheat	Scrambled Eggs w/ Mushrooms, Onion & Salsa Bacon	Two Eggs Sausage Bell Peppers	Buckwheat	Buckwheat
Snack	One Apple	One Cup of Fruit Salad	One Cup of Cantaloupe	10-12 Grapes	One Banana 1 Tbsp Cashew Butter	One Cup of Fresh Pineapple	One Cup of Fruit Salad
Lunch	Deli Meat Carrots Tomatoes Green Salad	Chicken Kabobs Rapini Squash & Zucchini	Deli Meat Carrots Tomatoes Green Salad	Pork Roast Baked Sweet Potatoes Green Beans Green Salad	Deli Meat Carrots Tomatoes Green Salad	Steak Baby Red Beets Spinach	Scrambled Eggs w/ Mushrooms, Onion & Salsa Sausage Spinach
Snack	Hot Lemon-water One Peach	Hot Lemon-water	Hot Lemon-water 8-10 Cherries	Hot Lemon-water One Cup of Cantaloupe	Hot Lemon-water One Cup of Fresh Pineapple	Hot Lemon-water	Hot Lemon-water 8-10 Cherries
Dinner	Chicken Kabobs Rapini Squash & Zucchini	Salmon Fillet Asparagus Swiss Chard	Pork Roast Baked Sweet Potatoes Green Beans Green Salad	Scallop Stir Fry Broccoli Carrots	Steak Baby Red Beets Spinach	Scrambled Eggs w/ Mushrooms, Onion & Salsa Sausage Spinach	Grilled Chicken Breast Grated Zucchini & Red Onion Kale
Snack	One Cup of Fruit Salad	5-6 Strawberries	One Peach	Hot Lemon-water	One Orange	One Cup of Fruit Salad	One Peach

Grocery List Month 2 - Week 4

Meats
Deli Meat
Skinless Chicken Breasts
Salmon Fillets
Pork Roast
Scallops
Steak
Bacon
Sausage

Vegetables
Bell Peppers (Yellow, Red, Orange)
Tomatoes
Carrots
Green Salad
Rapini
Yellow Squash
Zucchini
Avocado
Asparagus
Swiss Chard
Sweet Potatoes (yams)
Green Beans
Mushrooms (small Portobello)
Broccoli
Spinach
Onion (Purple and yellow)
Baby Red Beets
Kale
Cascading Farms Stir Fry Vegetables, frozen
Garlic

Fruit
Apples
Peaches/Nectarines
Lemons
Strawberries

Pineapple
Blueberries
Mangos
Grapes
Cantaloupe
Bananas
Oranges

Misc.
Eggs
Butter
Nut Butter (Cashew, Almond, or Peanut)
Olive Oil
Skewers
Parchment Paper

Spices
Ground Coriander
Red pepper flakes
Celtic Sea Salt
Cayenne Pepper

Recipes – Month 2 - Week 4

Chicken Kabobs
This recipe was taken from *The Fat Flush Plan by* Ann Louise Gittleman
1lb of skinless, boneless chicken breast cut into 1-inch cubes
2 cups of zucchini, cubed
2 cups yellow squash, cubed
2 cups of red pepper, cubed
½ lb of small Portobello mushrooms
2 cups of purple onions, cubed
Lemon wedges, for garnish

Preheat grill or broiler
Alternate chicken and vegetable cubes on skewers
Grill for about 15-20 minutes, turning at least once until chicken is cooked through
Remove from the grill onto a serving platter.
Garnish with lemon wedges.
Makes 4 Servings

Rapini
Wash the Rapini and shake off the water. Cut off the heavier stem bottoms. Blanch in boiling water for one minute. Drain and dry, then sauté in butter over medium heat. Add minced garlic for extra flavor.

Salmon Fillet
Ask for skinless salmon if you are going to cook in a skillet. This is great over medium heat in butter, fresh lemon juice, and minced garlic.

Swiss chard
Cut the stalks away from the leaf. Cut stalks into 1-inch pieces, sauté in butter or coconut oil over low heat for 15 minutes or until tender. Add strips of chard leaves. Cook over medium heat until wilted.

Pork Roast
This is best cooked in a crock-pot. Add ½ - 1 cup of beef broth and about 3 Tbsp of coconut oil or butter to keep moist. Cook on low heat for about 4 hours for 2-3 lbs. You can also add cayenne pepper, basil, or stuff with garlic cloves and rosemary.

Green Beans with Mushrooms
Green beans
Bacon, Mushrooms

Wash and cut ends off of green beans
Cut bacon into small pieces and cook in a skillet
Add green beans and cook until tender about 15-20 minutes

Add mushrooms and cook until tender

Baked Sweet Potato

Preheat the oven to 400 degrees. Pierce Sweet Potato with a fork. Rub outside with generous amounts of butter. Wrap in parchment paper and bake until tender (about 1 ½ hours for a medium potatoes).

Scallop Stir Fry

1 lb Scallops, wash and trimmed
2 bags of Cascading Farms stir fry vegetables, frozen
¼ cup butter or olive oil
¼ tsp red pepper flakes
½ tsp Celtic sea salt
Juice from ½ of a large lemon

Melt butter or coconut oil in a wok or large skillet. When the vegetable have thawed and are beginning to soften, add scallops, red pepper flakes, and Celtic sea salt. Cook until scallops are opaque and add lemon juice. Serve immediately!

Baby Red Beets

Wash beets and cut away greens. Remove skins. Steam for about 30 minutes or until soft. Add butter before serving for a little extra flavor.

Grated Zucchini & Purple Onion

2 large Zucchini, grated
½ Purple Onion, grated
½ tsp coriander
2 cloves of garlic, minced
¼ cup butter

Melt butter in a skillet. Add zucchini, red onion, coriander, and garlic. Cook over medium – high heat; sauté the zucchini mixture until it browns.

MONTH 3
MENUS, GROCERY LISTS AND RECIPES
Dietary Restrictions:

_____

_____

_____

_____

_____

_____

_____

Suggested Substitutions:

_____

_____

_____

_____

_____

_____

MONTH 3, WEEK 1 MENU

	Monday	Tuesday	Wednesday	Thursday	Friday	Saturday	Sunday
Breakfast	Two Eggs Sautéed Spinach and Tomatoes	Scrambled Eggs w/ Mushrooms &Onions	Cream of Buckwheat	Two Eggs Bacon Bell Pepper	Two Eggs Bacon Asparagus	Two Eggs Sliced Turkey Sliced Tomatoes Avocado	Cream of Buckwheat
Snack	One Banana Cashew Butter	One Orange	Cashew Butter	Fruit Salad	8-12 Cherries	Cashew Butter	10-12 Grapes
Lunch	Sliced Turkey Salad (lettuce, tomatoes, baby carrots) Olive Oil Lemon Juice	Tuna Fish Salad Salad (lettuce, carrots, bell pepper)	Grilled Pork Chops Golden Beets Broccoli	Cabbage and Beef Cauliflower	Rosemary & Garlic Roast Carrots Tomatoes	Grilled Chicken Breast Squash Zucchini Red Beets	Meat Loaf Green Beans Salad Lemon Juice Olive Oil
Snack	Hot Lemon-water 12 Grapes	Hot Lemon-water 8-12 Cherries	Hot Lemon-water One Cup of Fresh Pineapple Chunks	Hot Lemon-water 12 Grapes	Hot Lemon-water	Hot Lemon-water	Hot Lemon-water
Dinner	Tuna Fish Salad Salad (lettuce, carrots, bell pepper, walnuts) Olive Oil Lemon Juice	Grilled Pork Chops Golden Beets Broccoli	Cabbage and Beef Cauliflower	Rosemary & Garlic Roast Asparagus Carrots	Grilled Chicken Breast Squash Zucchini Red Beets	Meat Loaf Green Beans Sweet Potato Chips	Veggie Omelet (mushrooms, onion, artichoke hearts, tomatoes) Sliced Turkey
Snack	4-5 Strawberries	One Apple	Fruit Salad	One Orange	10-12 Grapes	Fruit Salad	1 Tbsp Cashew Butter

Grocery List – Month 3 - Week 1

Meats
Sliced Turkey
Pork Chops
Ground Beef
Chicken Breasts
Bacon
Tuna Fish
Beef Roast

Vegetables
Onions
Bell Peppers (Green, Yellow, Red, and Orange)
Spinach
Tomatoes – Large
Tomatoes – Grape
Mushrooms
Asparagus
Golden Baby Beets
Red Baby Beets
Baby Carrots (peeled, cut)
Baby Carrots (unpeeled and uncut)
Broccoli
Cabbage
Cauliflower
Lettuce
Sweet Potatoes (Jewel or Garnet Yams)
Squash
Zucchini
Artichoke Hearts - Canned
Rotel Tomatoes
Green Beans
Celery
Parsley
Garlic
Avocados

Fruit
Bananas
Fresh Pineapple

Cherries
Grapes
Oranges
Blueberries
Raspberries
Strawberries

Misc.
Butter – Unsalted Sweet Cream
Eggs
Cashew Butter
Olive Oil
Beef Broth
Cream of Buckwheat
Grade B Maple Syrup
Walnuts or Almonds
Dill Relish
Mayonnaise
No-Salt-Added Glen Muir Tomato Sauce

Spices
Celtic Sea Salt
Cayenne Pepper
Rosemary – fresh

Recipes- Month 3, Week 1

Traditional Tuna Fish Salad

2 6-oz cans of Tuna Fish (packed in spring water)
2 Tbsp of dill relish
1 Tbsp of Mayonnaise
4 Soft Boiled Eggs, chopped
Salt and Pepper to desired taste
¼ Medium yellow onion, chopped (optional)

Mix all ingredients in a large bowl.
Makes 4 servings

Cabbage and Beef

16 ounces (1 pound) of ground beef
1 large head of green cabbage, shredded
1 can of Rotel Tomatoes
1 large yellow onion, chopped
Salt and Pepper
Cayenne Pepper (optional)

Brown ground beef and onion in a skillet.
Place shredded cabbage, tomatoes, onion, and ground beef in a large pot and cook over medium heat for approximately 30 minutes.
Add salt, pepper, and cayenne pepper for desired taste.
Makes 4 Servings

Garlic and Rosemary Beef Roast

2 ½ pound beef roast
8-10 cloves of garlic, peeled
Fresh Rosemary
1 cup of beef broth

Make small slits in the beef roast and stuff with garlic cloves and fresh rosemary on both sides
Place roast in crock pot and pour beef broth over roast
Set the crock pot on low heat for 6 hours
Makes 8-9 servings

Cream of Buckwheat

You can buy this at Whole Foods or Wild Oats. Prepare as directed on the container. It is very easy to get creative with oatmeal. You can add butter, fruit, Grade B Maple Syrup, or RAW nuts. Just remember the rules: No Sugar or Dairy!!!

Yummy Meatloaf

(Taken from *The Fat Flush Plan by* Louise Gittleman)

16 ounces of ground beef
1 c spinach, chopped
1 c onion, diced
4 garlic cloves, minced
½ teaspoon cayenne pepper (optional)
4 tsp fresh parsley, chopped
4 tbsp no-salt-added Muir Glen Tomato Sauce

Preheat oven to 400 degrees
Place the meat, spinach, onion, garlic, cayenne, and parsley in the bowl of a food processor and blend.
Press into a loaf pan (or square glass pan) and glaze the top with the tomato sauce
Bake for approximately 45 minutes.
Makes 4 servings

Sweet Potato Chips

2 long, skinny jewel yams
½ stick of butter

Pre-heat oven to 400 degrees
Peel yams and slice into 1/8 of and inch rounds
Spread evenly onto a rimmed baking sheet
Cut butter into 4 equal pieces and place on top of yams
Stir every 10 minutes for 30-45 minutes (depending on desired crisp)
Makes 4 servings

Fruit Salad

This is very easy. Select 3 or 4 of your favorite fresh fruits. Cut into bite size pieces and squeeze ½ of a fresh lemon to prevent browning and it's ready to eat.

1 cup = 1 serving
Warning: measure out a serving before eating; it's easy to overeat!!!!!

All of the vegetables on the meal plan for this week taste wonderful when sautéed in butter with minced garlic. These include: asparagus, carrots, and broccoli. I usually steam the squash, zucchini, and cauliflower then add melted butter and garlic before serving.

MONTH 3, WEEK 2 MENU

	Monday	Tuesday	Wednesday	Thursday	Friday	Saturday	Sunday
Breakfast	Two Eggs Bacon Bell Pepper	Two Eggs w/Salsa Bacon Spinach	Oatmeal	Two Eggs Tomatoes Avocado	Scrambled Eggs w/ Mushrooms, Onion, Garlic & Spinach	Oatmeal	Two Eggs Bacon Bell Pepper
Snack	10-12 Grapes	One Apple	5-6 Strawberries	Fruit Salad	One Cup of Fresh Pineapple	One Banana	One Orange
Lunch	Deli Meat Grape Tomatoes Baby Carrots	Taco Salad Guacamole	Blackened Salmon Napa Cabbage Mashed Navy Beans w/ Garlic	Steak Blasted Sweet Potatoes Asparagus	Chicken Breast Roasted Broccoli Carrots	Artichoke, Sun-dried Tomatoes & Asparagus Egg Scramble Spinach	Stuffed Onion Casserole
Snack	Hot Lemon-water One Orange	Hot Lemon-water One Banana	Hot Lemon-water One Cup of Fresh Pineapple	Hot Lemon-water 1-2 Tbsp Nut-Butter	Hot Lemon-water 5 Strawberries	Hot Lemon-water One Apple	Hot Lemon-water 10-12 Grapes
Dinner	Taco Salad	Blackened Salmon Napa Cabbage Mashed Navy Beans w/ Garlic	Steak Blasted Sweet Potatoes Asparagus	Chicken Breast Roasted Broccoli Carrots	Artichoke, Sun-dried Tomatoes & Asparagus Egg Scramble Spinach	Stuffed Onion Casserole	Shepherd's Pie Green Beans w/ Stewed Tomatoes
Snack	One Apple	One Orange	Fruit Salad	10-12 Grapes	One Banana	Fruit Salad	1-2 Tbsp Nut Butter

104

Grocery List – Month 3 - Week 2

Meat
Ground Beef
Chicken Breasts
Salmon
Steak
Deli Meat
Bacon

Vegetables
Cauliflower
Garlic
Green onions (chives)
Cilantro
Black olives, canned, pitted
Carrots
Mushrooms
Bell Peppers (Green, yellow, & red)
Onions
Jalapeños
Parsley
Sweet Potatoes
Napa Cabbage
Avocados
Green Leaf Lettuce
Large tomato
Grape Tomatoes
Snow Peas
Spinach
Green Beans
Asparagus
Artichoke Hearts, canned
Sun-dried Tomatoes
Navy Beans, canned

Fruit
Apples
Bananas
Strawberries
Pineapples

Peaches
Oranges
Blueberries
Grapes
Lemons
Limes

Misc.
Nut butter (Cashew or Almond)
Olive Oil
Apple cider Vinegar
Malt Vinegar
Butter
Eggs
Refried Beans
Salsa
Pico de Gallo
Dry white wine (optional) Sauvignon
Blanc, Chenin Blanc, or Chablis
Sesame Seeds
Chicken Broth
Beef Broth
Stevia Plus
Muir Glen Tomato Puree
Muir Glen Tomato Sauce
Muir Glen Diced Tomatoes

Spices
Onion Powder
Garlic Powder
Cayenne Pepper
Celtic Sea Salt
Freshly ground pepper
Chili Powder

Recipes – Month 3 - Week 2

Taco Salad (without the taco!)
2 lbs of ground beef,
2 tsp chili powder
2 head of green leaf lettuce, cut into small pieces
2 large tomato, diced
2 can of refried beans (optional)
Salsa or Pico de Gallo
Guacamole
Brown ground beef and add chili powder
Layer refried beans and beef onto a plate
Then add lettuce, tomatoes, salsa or Pico de Gallo, and guacamole.
*(Refried beans are **not** optimal for weight loss. The carbohydrate to protein ratio is really high. If you are trying to lose weight eliminate the refried beans.)
Makes 8 servings

Guacamole
4-5 Soft Avocados, peeled and seeded
3 cloves of garlic, minced
3 tbsp of cilantro, chopped
The juice from one small lime
¼ cup of Salsa or Pico de Gallo
1 tsp of Celtic sea salt
2-3 tbsp jalapeños, chopped (optional)
Mash avocados
Add garlic, cilantro, lime juice, salsa or Pico de Gallo, and sea salt
Mix together
If you like guacamole more spicy add jalapeños

Blackened Salmon on Zesty Cabbage
From Simply *Shrimp, Salmon, and Steaks by Leslie Pendleton*
1 Onion, sliced thin
¼ cup butter
1 tsp grated lemon zest
3 tbsp fresh lemon juice
1 cup dry white wine (optional) ex. Sauvignon blanc, Chenin blanc, or Chablis
1 small head Napa cabbage, sliced thin crosswise
4 tsp chili powder
4 tsp sesame seeds
2 tsp salt
1 tsp black pepper
1 tbsp butter or same amount of coconut oil

1 ½ lbs center-cut salmon fillet, skinned and cut crosswise into 4 portion

In a large skillet, cook the onion in the ¼ cup of butter over moderate heat, stirring occasionally, until pale golden. Add the lemon zest, juice, wine, and cook over moderately high heat until liquid is reduced by half, about 15 minutes. Add the cabbage and cook, stirring until it is wilted and just tender. Add salt and pepper to taste and keep warm while the salmon is cooking. In a small bowl, combine chili powder, sesame seeds, salt, and pepper. Coat the salmon with the mixture. Heat 1 tbsp of butter in a large nonstick skillet over moderately high heat and add the salmon. If the salmon is browning too quickly, reduce the heat to moderate.   Cook for four to five minutes on each side or until brown and crisp and just cooked through.
Divide the cabbage among four plates and top with the salmon.

Mashed White Beans and Garlic
From Simply *Shrimp, Salmon, and Steaks by Leslie Pendleton.*
1 19-ounce can white navy beans
2 large cloves of garlic, minced
2 tbsp olive oil
1-2 cup chicken broth
Freshly ground black pepper
Nu-Salt

Drain the beans in a colander and rinse well.
In a saucepan, cook the garlic in oil over moderately low heat until softened, about 5 minutes.
Add the broth and beans and simmer for 5 minutes. Mash the mixture with a potato masher or transfer to a food processor or blender and puree until just smooth. Season with pepper and salt

Blasted Sweet Potatoes
From Simply *Shrimp, Salmon, and Steaks by* Leslie Pendleton
2 ½ lbs sweet potatoes, peeled
3 tbsp olive oil
4 tbsp malt vinegar
1 tsp Celtic sea salt
3 tbsp minced fresh parsley
Freshly ground black pepper

Preheat oven to 475 degrees.
Cut the sweet potatoes into ½ inch dice. On a large rimmed baking sheet, toss the potato cube with the oil until they are well coated. Roast the potatoes in the oven, turning them occasionally, for 20-30 minutes. The potatoes will be tender long before they are crisp, so cook until they are deep golden but do not let them burn. Transfer the potatoes to a bowl and toss with the vinegar. Add Nu-salt, parsley, and pepper and toss. Serve immediately
Serves 4-6

Stuffed Onion Casserole
From *The Fat Flush Cookbook by* Ann Louise Gittleman

4 extra large onions, peeled, cut in half crosswise, with centers removed and three layers of onion still intact
1 green pepper, chopped
1 lb ground beef
1 egg beaten
1 tsp garlic powder
Handful of fresh cilantro, chopped
1 cup Hearty Barbecue Sauce

Preheat oven to degrees. Blanch onion halves in hot water and set aside. Chop the onion centers to make ¾ cup. Combine chopped onion, green pepper, ground beef, egg, garlic powder, cilantro, and ½ cup Hearty Barbecue Sauce. Mix well and make 4 large meatballs. Stuff meatballs into the four onion halves and place the top half of the onion over the meatball making sure there is a gap between the top and bottom of the onion. Place stuffed onions into a shallow baking dish and bake for 50-60 minutes. Baste with the remaining barbecue sauce the last 15 minutes of baking.
Makes 4 servings.

Hearty Barbecue Sauce:
From *The Fat Flush Cookbook by* Ann Louise Gittleman
½ cup of onion, finely chopped
2 garlic cloves, minced
2 tablespoons plus1/4 cup beef broth
¼ cup apple cider vinegar
1 teaspoon onion powder
½ teaspoon Stevia Plus
1 8-ounce can no-salt-added Muir Glen Tomato Puree'
1 teaspoon cayenne, or to taste
½ jalapeño, seeded and minced

Sauté onion and garlic in 2 tablespoons broth until tender. Add remaining broth, vinegar, onion powder, Stevia Plus, tomato puree', cayenne, and jalapeño. Bring to a boil, reduce heat, and simmer for about 30 minutes. Cool and store in the fridge.

Yields about 1 cup

Sheppard's Pie
From *The Fat Flush Cookbook by* Ann Louise Gittleman
1 pound lean ground beef
1 medium onion, chopped
4 garlic cloves, minced
1 green pepper, chopped
8 ounces mushrooms, slice
1-teaspoon cayenne
½ teaspoon onion powder

110

½ teaspoon garlic powder

2 small carrots, grated

12 black olives, pitted and chopped

Handful of fresh cilantro, chopped

1 8-ounce can no salt added tomato sauce

1 14 1/2 ounce can no salt added diced tomato

2 cups mashed cauliflower, see recipe

Preheat oven to 350 degrees F. In a large, nonstick skillet, brown ground beef, onion, and garlic. When beef is nearly done, add green pepper, mushrooms, cayenne, onion powder, and garlic powder. When beef is no longer pink, transfer to a large casserole dish. Add carrots, olives, cilantro, tomato sauce, and diced tomatoes to a casserole dish and mix well. Spread mashed cauliflower over the top.

Bake in the oven for 30 minutes. Place under broiler for 3 minutes or until browned on top.

Marvelously Mashed Cauliflower
From *The Fat Flush Cookbook by* Ann Louise Gittleman

1 medium head cauliflower, cut into florets

1 cup purified water

2 garlic cloves, minced

1 teaspoon fresh chives, chopped

½ teaspoon onion powder

½ teaspoon fresh parsley, chopped

1 tablespoon Chicken or Beef broth

In a medium pot, place cauliflower with water and bring to a quick boil. Lower heat to simmer and cover. Cook for an additional 12 minutes or until soft. Drain, transfer cauliflower to a bowl, and mash. Blend in garlic, chives, onion powder, parsley, and broth with the mashed cauliflower. Serve Hot. Please note you may want to use a food processor to mash the cauliflower or a potato masher will work just fine.

MONTH 3, WEEK 3 MENU

	Monday	Tuesday	Wednesday	Thursday	Friday	Saturday	Sunday
Breakfast	Scrambled Eggs w/ Salsa Spinach	Cream of Buckwheat	Two Soft Boiled Eggs Sliced Tomatoes Avocados	Two Eggs Bell Peppers Spinach Broccoli	Cream of Buckwheat	Cream of Buckwheat	Two Eggs Bacon Asparagus Tomatoes
Snack	One Mango	One Apple	10-12 Grapes	Fruit Salad	One egg	One Plum	Fruit Salad
Lunch	Shepherd's Pie Green Beans w/ Stewed Tomatoes	Tuna Fish Salad Bed of Greens Fresh Lemon Juice	Tarragon Turkey Burgers Shredded Zucchini Green Salad Emerald Greens Salad Dressing	Slow Cooker Beef Stew Green Salad Emerald Greens Dressing	Stuffed Cabbage Brussel Sprouts Carrots	Salmon Patties Asparagus Sautéed Eggplant	Mushroom, Onion, Garlic & Salsa Egg Scramble Broccoli
Snack	Hot Lemon-water 5 Strawberries	Hot Lemon-water One Plum	Hot Lemon-water One Banana	Hot Lemon-water One Orange	Hot Lemon-water One Cup of Fresh Pineapple Chunks	Hot Lemon-water One Mango	Hot Lemon-water Two Kiwis
Dinner	Tuna Fish Salad Bed of Greens Fresh Lemon Juice	Tarragon Turkey Burgers Shredded Zucchini Green Salad Emerald Greens Salad Dressing	Slow Cooker Beef Stew Green Salad Emerald Greens Dressing	Stuffed Cabbage Brussel Sprouts Carrots	Salmon Patties Asparagus Sautéed Eggplant	Mushroom, Onion, Garlic & Salsa Egg Scramble Broccoli	Grilled Chicken Sweet Potato Chips Spinach
Snack	10-12 Grapes	One Orange	Fruit Salad	2 Tbsp Nut Butter	One Grapefruit	Fruit Salad	One Banana One Tbsp Nut Butter

Grocery List –Month 3 - Week 3

Meat
Tuna Fish
Ground Turkey
Stew Meat
Ground Beef
Salmon Fillet
Chicken breast
Bacon &/or Sausage

Vegetables
Spinach
Mixed Salad Greens
Zucchini
Red/Purple onion
Yellow Onions
Bell Pepper (green, yellow, red)
Roma Tomatoes
Large Tomatoes
Scallions
Cauliflower
Broccoli
Carrots
Cabbage
Leeks
Ginger
Garlic
Parsley
Brussel Sprouts
Dill, Fresh
Asparagus
Eggplant
Mushrooms
Sweet Potatoes
Avocados

Fruit
Mangos
Strawberries
Lemons
Grapes

Apples
Plums
Bananas
Oranges
Pineapple
Kiwi
Grapefruit

Misc.
Eggs
Butter
Salsa
Cream of Buckwheat
Nut Butter
Mayonnaise
Dijon Mustard
Flaxseed Oil
Apple Cider Vinegar
Beef Broth

Spices
Salt
Pepper
Tarragon, fresh or dried
Coriander
Dill, dried
Cayenne Pepper
Cumin
Fennel, dried
Cinnamon, ground
Turmeric, ground
Whole cloves

Recipes-Month 3, Week 3

Healthy Tuna Salad
2 12-ounce cans Tuna Fish, drained
1 cup Red Grapes, washed and halved
1 cup baby spinach leaves, washed and chopped
¼ cup purple onion, finely chopped
2 Tbsp mayonnaise
Salt and pepper to taste

Mix all ingredients together. Serve over a bed of mixed salad greens.

TARRAGON TURKEY BURGER
1 lb free-range ground turkey breast
1/2 c. coarsely shredded zucchini (or celery)
1/4 c. chopped red onion
1 Tbsp fresh or dried tarragon leaves
2 tsp Dijon mustard
1/2 tsp sea salt
3 grinds of fresh black pepper
3 large eggs

Preheat broiler. In mixing bowl, combine ground turkey with
zucchini, red onion, tarragon, mustard, Spike, pepper, and eggs. Mix
thoroughly.
Shape into patties. Place on broiler pan. Broil 5 minutes onto a
side until browned. Served immediately.

Serves 4: Preparation time = 5 min.

Grated Zucchini & Purple Onion
2 large Zucchini, grated
½ Purple Onion, grated
½ tsp coriander
2 cloves of garlic, minced
¼ cup butter

Melt butter in a skillet. Add zucchini, red onion, coriander, and garlic. Cook over medium – high heat;
sauté the zucchini mixture until it browns.

Emerald Greens Dressing
From *The Fat Flush Plan By* Ann Louise Gittleman

115

You need enough dressing for two dinners and two lunches. This recipe only makes about ¾ cup so you will probably need to double or triple the recipe.

4 Tbsp Flaxseed Oil
1 Tbsp Apple Cider Vinegar
4 Tbsp Green Pepper, chopped
½ tsp dried dill
1 Tbsp fresh parsley, chopped
1 Tbsp onion, chopped

Place all ingredients into a small jar and shake vigorously. Serve immediately or store in the refrigerator for up to 4 days.
Makes ¾ cup

Slow Cooker Beef Stew
From *The Fat Flush Plan By* Ann Louise Gittleman

1 ½ pounds stew meat, lean, and trimmed of all visible fat, cut into chunks

4 Roma tomatoes, cut into chunks
2 scallions, thinly sliced
1 teaspoon Fat Flush Curry Seasoning
1 teaspoon cayenne
1 small head cauliflower, cut into florets
1 small head broccoli, cut into florets
1 carrot, grated
1 cup purified water

Mix all ingredients in a 3 ½ quart or larger slow cooker. Cover and cook on low for 6 to 8 hours until beef is cooked through and vegetables are tender.

Fat Flush Curry Seasoning

4 tablespoons ground coriander
1 tablespoon ground cumin
1 tablespoon dried fennel
1 tablespoon cayenne
1 tablespoon ground cinnamon
1 ½ teaspoons ground turmeric
5 whole cloves

Crush all the ingredients together using a mortar and pestle or grind together in a food processor until fine. Store in an airtight container in the refrigerator or in a cool, dry place away from heat and moisture.

Stuffed Cabbage
From *The Fat Flush Plan By* Ann Louise Gittleman

8 Large Cabbage leaves, washed, ¼ cup leeks, finely chopped
1 tsp fresh ginger, grated or a pinch of dried ginger, ½ lb ground beef
2 Garlic cloves, minced, 1 egg lightly beaten
2 cups beef broth
8 toothpicks
2 tbsp fresh parsley

In a large pot, cook cabbage in boiling water until it becomes soft enough to be used as wrapping. Gently remove the cabbage from the hot water with a slotted spoon, refresh in cold water, and dry. In a medium skillet, sauté leek, ginger, beef, and garlic until the beef is cooked through. Add the egg to the meat and mix thoroughly for filling. Divide the filling into 8 portions, placing each portion in the middle of the cabbage leaf. Fold the two opposite sides of the leaf over the filling and roll up tightly, securing the toothpicks. Arrange the cabbage rolls in the skillet, add broth, and simmer for 20 minutes. Sprinkle with parsley.
Makes 2 servings.

Salmon Cakes
Taken from *the Fat Flush Cookbook by* Ann Louise Gittleman

8 oz cooked salmon fillet
½ cup scallions, finely chopped
2 tsp fresh dill
2 garlic cloves, minced
Splash of fresh lemon juice
1 egg, beaten
Preheat the oven to 350 degrees. Place salmon in a large bowl and separate with a fork. Mix in scallions, dill, garlic, lemon juice, and egg. Shape mixture into two patties, about ¾ inch thick. Place patties in a nonstick baking dish or nonstick baking sheet in the oven. Bake in the oven for about 15 minutes or until golden brown and cooked through.
Makes 2 servings

Sautéed Eggplant
2 Medium Eggplants, peeled and diced
½ cup butter
Sauté in a large skillet for about 15-20 minutes or until tender.

MONTH 3, WEEK 4 MENU

	Monday	Tuesday	Wednesday	Thursday	Friday	Saturday	Sunday
Breakfast	2 Eggs Spinach Bell Pepper	2 Eggs Tomatoes Avocados	2 Eggs w/ Pico de Gallo & spinach Bacon or Sausage	Cream of Buckwheat	Cream of Buckwheat	2 Eggs Bacon or Sausage Asparagus w/ Mushrooms	Cream of Buckwheat
Snack	5-6 Strawberries	Fruit Salad	1 cup Pineapple	1 Banana	1 cup Berries	Fruit Salad	1 Plum
Lunch	Grilled Chicken Sweet Potato Chips Spinach	Grilled Pork Chops Carrots Green Cabbage w/ Pico de Gallo	2 Soft Boiled Eggs Green Salad Tomatoes Carrots	Ground Beef w/ onions, mushrooms, & cayenne pepper Green Beans Sweet Potato Chips	Chicken Kabobs Sautéed Eggplant Red Swiss Chard	Artichoke heart, sun-dried tomato, & onion egg scramble Bacon Avocado	Steak Asparagus Broccoli Cauliflower
Snack	1 Banana	1 Orange	10-12 Grapes	1 Pear	1 Orange	1 Plum	10-12 Grapes
Dinner	Grilled Pork Chops Carrots Green Cabbage w/ Pico de Gallo	Salmon Fillet Brussel Sprouts Red Baby Beets	Ground Beef w/ onions, mushrooms, & cayenne pepper Green Beans Sweet Potato Chips	Chicken Kabobs Sautéed Eggplant Red Swiss Chard	Artichoke heart, sun-dried tomato, & onion egg scramble Bacon Avocado	Steak Asparagus Broccoli Cauliflower	Grilled Chicken Breasts over green salad w/ carrots, shredded beets, bell pepper, avocado, & chopped almonds.
Snack	Fruit Salad	1 Pear	5-6 Strawberries	10-12 Grapes	Fruit Salad	1 Banana	Serve w/ lemon juice or coconut oil and balsamic vinegar

Grocery List – Month 3 - Week 4

Meat
Bacon or Sausage
Chicken Breasts
Steak
Ground Beef
Pork Chops

Vegetables
Spinach
Bell Peppers
Sweet Potatoes
Carrots
Green Cabbage
Tomatoes
Avocados
Brussel Sprouts
Red Baby Beets
Green Salad
Green Beans
Mushrooms
Onions, Purple and yellow
Eggplant
Red Swiss chard
Artichoke Hearts (canned)
Sun Dried Tomatoes (usu. located in the olive bar)
Asparagus
Broccoli
Cauliflower
Zucchini
Yellow Squash

Fruit
Bananas
Pineapples
Berries
Strawberries
Plums
Pears

Oranges
Grapes
Lemons

Spices
Cayenne Pepper
Sea Salt "a pinch"
Pepper

Misc.
Olive Oil
Balsamic Vinegar
Almonds
Pico de Gallo
Eggs
Butter
Spaghetti sauce (Muir Glen)

Recipes – Month 3 - Week 4

This week there aren't many recipes. Grill the meat on a grill or broil in the oven. Sauté the vegetables in butter, or steam them and then add melted butter and garlic.

Green Cabbage

1 Medium head of cabbage, shredded
1 – 1 ½ cups of Pico de Gallo
Add all ingredients and sauté over medium heat until cabbage begins to brown. Serve immediately.
Serves 4

Salmon Fillet

1 lb Salmon Fillet, skinned
Sauté in a skillet with lemon juice and butter for about 7 minutes. Add minced Garlic and cook for an additional 3-5 minutes.
Serves 2

Brussel Sprouts

20-30 Brussel Sprouts, washed, cut into halves, and outer layer peeled
3 Tbsp butter
Sauté Brussel sprouts until soft and beginning to brown.
Serves 4

Red Baby Beets

8 Red Baby Beets, peeled
Steam for approximately 30 minutes or until tender
Serves 4

Ground Beef

2 lbs Ground Beef
1 Medium Onion, chopped
2 Cups sliced mushrooms
2 cups Spaghetti Sauce (Muir Glen)
½ tsp cayenne pepper
Brown ground beef, onions, and cayenne pepper. Drain grease. Add mushrooms and spaghetti sauce. Cook over medium - low heat for an additional 15-20 minutes.

Green Beans

4-6 Strips of bacon, cut into small pieces
2 lbs green beans, washed with ends removed
Nu-Salt, to taste

Cayenne pepper, to taste

Cook bacon over medium heat for approximately 5 minutes or until it becomes brown. Add green beans and cook covered over medium heat for 15 minutes or until tender. Stir every couple of minutes to avoid bacon burning. Add salt and cayenne pepper to taste.

Serves 4

Sweet Potato Chips

2 Yams (longer yams are easier to cut), peeled and cut into 1/8 inch rounds

1/3 cup of butter

Preheat oven to 385 degrees. Place yams and butter on a rimmed cookie sheet and cook for 1 hour or until desired crispness. Turning yams every 5-7 minutes allows even cooking.

Serves 4

Chicken Kabobs

This recipe was taken from *The Fat Flush Plan by* Ann Louise Gittleman

1lb of skinless, boneless chicken breast cut into 1-inch cubes

2 cups of zucchini, cubed

2 cups yellow squash, cubed

2 cups of red pepper, cubed

½ lb of small Portobello mushrooms

2 cups of purple onions, cubed

Lemon wedges, for garnish

Preheat grill or broiler

Alternate chicken and vegetable cubes on skewers

Grill for about 15-20 minutes, turning at least once, until chicken is cooked through

Remove from the grill onto a serving platter.

Garnish with lemon wedges

Makes 4 Servings

Eggplant

2 Medium eggplants, diced

3-4 Tbsp butter

Sauté eggplant in butter for about 10 minutes or until browned.

s

Red Swiss chard

2 bunches of Swiss chard (red, green, or rainbow), washed

2 Tbsp butter

Remove center rib from the leaf. Cut into 1-2 inch pieces. Cut leaves into bite size pieces. Sauté center rib in butter first until just tender. Add leaves and sauté until wilted.

Serves 4

Fruit Salad

This is very easy. Select 3 or 4 of your favorite fresh fruits. Cut into bite size pieces and squeeze ½ of a fresh lemon to prevent browning and it's ready to eat.

1 cup = 1 serving
Warning: measure out a serving before eating; it's easy to overeat!!!!!

NOTES:

Endnotes/Sources

has the world's largest diabetes population (400 BC) diabetes